Acclaim for Jay Winner, M.D.'s
Take the Stress out of Your Life

"A great teaching, simply presented. It's practical, wise, and truly valuable for a healthy life."

—JACK KORNFIELD, PH.D., author of *A Path with Heart*

"*Take the Stress out of Your Life* is practical, useful, and effective."

—DEAN ORNISH, M.D., author of
Stress, Diet, and Your Heart and *Love and Survival*

"I highly recommend this book and CD set as a wonderful, easy way to decrease your stress and improve your health. It is an entertaining read packed with important and useful information."

—JACK CANFIELD, cocreator of the Chicken Soup for the Soul series

"There is genius in simplicity! [*Take the Stress out of Your Life*] is excellent. It is the best new book about stress management that I have read in years."

—RONALD G. NATHAN, PH.D., coauthor of
Stress Management: A Comprehensive Guide to Wellness

"This book is succinct, interesting, and well written. Nearly everyone will benefit from its practical techniques. This type of education helps patients and doctors better manage stress."

—RICHARD ROBERTS, M.D., J.D.,
past president of the American Academy of Family Physicians and
president–elect of the World Organization for Family Doctors

"Being a healthy person in today's world means knowing how to manage stress, and this resource is a must-have. Jay Winner has compiled a great book on everything you ever wanted to know about stress and how to live in joy!"

—CHERIE CARTER-SCOTT, PH.D.,
author of *If Life Is a Game, These Are the Rules*

D0465423

"A terrific guide—accessible and immensely practical—for dealing with the largest everyday problem of modern times. Dr. Winner makes a stress-free life seem within our reach. Honestly, I learned a lot myself!"

—DIANA WINSTON, director of Mindfulness Education, Mindful Awareness Research Center, UCLA, and author of *Wide Awake: A Buddhist Guide for Teens*

"Dr. Winner covers an amazing amount of material in a reasonably few number of pages. . . . His sincerity, honesty, and humility are compelling and his relaxed, conversational, anecdotal writing style renders this information accessible to everyone—including the type of person who would never read, much less enjoy, a book on stress management. . . . I will give [*Take the Stress out of Your Life*] to my patients because I trust they will enjoy it and therefore will be much more likely to follow its suggestions than most of the other stress management books I have read."

—LARRY BASCOM, PH.D., psychologist and past president of the Santa Barbara County Psychological Association

"Although there are now myriad resources about stress management, most either focus on one method or provide an overview that is either too esoteric or too simplistic. Dr. Winner has accomplished the significant task of integrating all of the major contributions to stress management in a very readable manner. His book provides thoughtful and pragmatic one-stop shopping for readers who wish to better manage stress and to improve the quality of their lives."

—STEVE SHEARER, PH.D., cofounder, Anxiety and Stress Disorders Institute of Maryland

"[A]n excellent antidote to the immense stresses of 21st century life as offered by author, medical doctor, and stress management instructor Jay Winner, M.D. From learning how to manage anger and frustration, to improving the quality of one's sleep, to simply better enjoying one's day, [*Take the Stress out of Your Life*] is an easy-to-read, 'reader friendly,' highly recommended addition to Self-Help reading lists, Self-Improvement reference library collections."

—MIDWEST BOOK REVIEW

"[A] useful, practical, and comprehensive guide for helping patients with stress reduction and improving the quality of their lives. Physicians and other health practitioners will find it an essential guide for group appointments and classes that support patients in behavioral changes that promote health on the spiritual, emotional, and physical levels. Patients will also find it readable and useful as a patient guide."

—LUCILLE MARCHAND, M.D., B.S.N.,
associate professor at the University of Wisconsin,
Department of Family Medicine, and integrative medicine
consultant at the UW Integrative Medicine Program

"Dr. Winner offers practical advice for dealing with everyday stress. You can use this book and CD set to help find personal peace in a chaotic world."

—BRUCE BAGLEY, M.D.,
past president of the American Academy of Family Physicians

"[*Take the Stress out of Your Life*] is understandable and engaging. It is written so that a layman can understand it, but it also provides physicians with the knowledge and skills they need to help patients manage stress."

—DAVID P. ZAJANO, M.D., chairman of the Department of
Family Practice, Franklin Square Hospital, and
past president of the Maryland Academy of Family Practice

"[*Take the Stress out of Your Life*] is an extremely important and effective tool for people dealing with stress and anxiety in our busy world."

—LYNN MATIS,
psychotherapist specializing in the treatment of anxiety

ABOUT THE AUTHOR

Jay Winner, M.D., is a family physician and stress expert who has helped thousands of patients deal with stress. He is the founder and director of the Stress Management Program for Sansum Clinic, one of California's largest medical clinics. Dr. Winner speaks on the topic of stress management to corporations, physician groups, counselors, military personnel, and government employees. He was the medical director of and a regular contributor to *Day-to-Day Health,* a national employee newsletter, and is quoted often as a stress expert in a wide variety of national print and electronic media. He lives in Santa Barbara, California, and is the chairman of the Department of Family Practice for Santa Barbara Cottage Hospital.

More information about him and his work is available at www.stressremedy.com.

Take the Stress out of Your Life

*A Medical Doctor's
Proven Program to
Minimize Stress and
Maximize Health*

JAY WINNER, M.D.

Da Capo
LIFE
LONG
A Member of the Perseus Books Group

Designed by Brent Wilcox

Library of Congress Cataloging-in-Publication Data
Winner, Jay.
    Take the stress out of your life : a medical doctor's proven program to minimize stress and maximize health / Jay Winner. — 1st Da Capo Press ed.
        p.   cm.
    Includes bibliographical references.
    ISBN 978-0-7382-1174-9 (alk. paper)
    1. Stress management.   2. Relaxation.   I. Title.
    RA785.W56 2008
    616.9'8—dc22

                                                        2007046821

First Da Capo Press edition 2008

Published by Da Capo Press
A Member of the Perseus Books Group
www.dacapopress.com

Da Capo Press books are available at special discounts for bulk purchases in the United States by corporations, institutions, and other organizations. For more information, please contact the Special Markets Department at the Perseus Books Group, 2300 Chestnut Street, Suite 200, Philadelphia, PA 19103, or call (800) 255-1514, or e-mail special.markets@perseusbooks.com.

1 2 3 4 5 6 7 8 9

*This book is dedicated to
my family, friends, patients, students, and teachers.*

CONTENTS

INTRODUCTION

Imagine a prehistoric man walking across a grassy savannah. Out of the corner of his eye, he sees a saber-toothed tiger stalking him. Boom! Instantly, hormones are released in the man's body that make his heart pound faster, his breath quicken, his pupils dilate, and his blood rush from his gut to his muscles. For the next few moments, as his body is flooded with extra oxygen and energy, he is stronger, faster, and sharper than normal. This reaction may well make the difference if he chooses to fight or (smarter still) flee the tiger. If the man is walking with a friend, and his friend's body does not have this "stress response," the friend is more likely to become lunch. But our prehistoric man wins the 50-yard dash and survives to pass his genes—and stress response—to future generations.

Today, we all have inherited this "fight-or-flight" response, which used to serve us so well. But we live in a vastly different world from that of our ancestors. The stress response evolved as a physical solution to a physical threat. Our world is still full of threats, but they are rarely physical ones, and physical responses are rarely appropriate. If your boss yells at you and you punch him in the nose, you'll get a pink slip. If you feel your blood pressure rising as you endure a traffic jam, and you respond by veering into the breakdown lane and flooring the gas pedal, you risk a ticket or even an accident.

The reality of the modern world is that, most of the time, the appropriate response to a stressful situation is simply to grin and bear it. And that's a problem. Because those stress hormones, triggered by ancient genes, still scream at us to do something physical. They cause real chemical and physical changes in the body as they shift all our systems to Code Red. The stressful tension created by that inner urgency, and the inability to act on it, isn't just uncomfortable. It exacerbates almost every type of illness you can think of. It can even kill. In one four-year study, caregivers with high levels of stress had a 63 percent greater risk of dying than people with normal stress. Another study showed that women under stress suffered actual changes in their DNA—the equivalent of aging 9 to 17 years. Still another found that men who had high surges in blood pressure due to stress had a 72 percent increased risk of stroke. Stress is implicated in everything from headaches and obesity to fibromyalgia, depression, and infertility. It erodes relationships and productivity. It will shorten your life and ruin your days. It is no laughing matter.

The bad news? There is no way to escape stress entirely. If you are an American adult, chances are almost 50/50 that you are feeling the debilitating effects of stress as you read these words. The chances are overwhelming that you will suffer from stress at some point in the future. Stress goes hand in hand with contemporary life. A small sampling of other illnesses it causes, or exacerbates, include heart disease, acne, eczema, psoriasis, irritable bowel syndrome, and heartburn. Stress may also affect the treatment of diabetes, high blood pressure, chronic pain, and asthma.

The good news? Probably no area of your health can be improved more easily, and with more beneficial impact, than stress. Manage your stress and you will worry less, live longer, and laugh more. Despite what you may have been led to believe, managing stress does not require years of study or learning any difficult or esoteric techniques. It is amazing how small changes in our thought patterns can cause large improvements in our ability to handle stress. Likewise, taking a few minutes to learn a basic 10-minute relaxation technique can pay off again and again. Even simple lifestyle changes will have a profound impact on stress. There is no single answer for dealing with stress, but there are numerous opportunities to control it.

That's what this book is about. Simply put, it is a stress management tool kit. Just as replacing a rock with a sledgehammer can turn an unworkable problem into a simple fix, having the right tools on hand for tackling stress can dispel what felt like an impossible burden. Not all tools will work for everyone. Depending on your personality and circumstances, you will find certain ideas and techniques that fit you best. Even if one chapter isn't helpful to you, please keep reading. One patient told me that the chapter on mindfulness changed her life, and another found that the chapter on communication skills made all the difference. But no matter who you are, you will find some techniques in this book that work. I know, because I've taught these techniques to thousands of people over the past fifteen years as director of the Stress Management Program at one of the largest medical clinics in California. I've even taught it to the staff at the clinic. I've seen firsthand the changes in how people enjoy their day and in how they get stuff done when they are relaxed and focused.

The funny thing is I didn't set out to become a stress specialist. I began my career doing regular family practice, but after less than a year of seeing patients, I saw in graphic detail that America had a major problem on its hands. My patients had physical ailments, sure, and they needed specific treatments for them, but in family practice I mostly treated people who were incredibly stressed-out. The more I talked with my patients—and I try to talk a lot with my patients, because I believe in treating the whole person—the more I realized that stress either was their primary problem or was aggravating their other concerns. These people didn't need more pills; they needed to learn how to unwind.

I wasn't the first doctor to recognize this problem. A recent survey showed that 97 percent of physicians are aware that stress often triggers or compounds patients' ailments. However, most doctors are too busy and stressed themselves to take the time to treat stress properly. It isn't unusual for a doctor to have all of 15 minutes to handle three different problems. Many doctors see 25 or 35 patients in one day. This isn't their choice, but they have to do the best they can under the circumstances. When a patient says, "My work is getting very stressful and now I have headaches every evening," the doctor may want to take two hours to do some stress management training and teach the patient some basic relaxation exercises, but that isn't an option. The patient wants fast relief, so the doctor says, "Here, take this medicine the next time you have a headache." Unfortunately, the basic problem has not been addressed.

Given the time constraints of a typical office visit, what alternatives does a family doctor have? In 1992, I decided to come up with a solution. There was no shortage of information. The questions of how to deal with stress and how to be happy have been around for thousands of years, and so have some of the best answers. From early in my training, I was aware of them and have been researching the answers for the past 30 years. I organized and led seminars in stress management for my patients and for other doctors' patients. I might not be able to do much for my patients' stress levels in one office visit, but if I could get them to take the stress management course, I could give them skills that would last a lifetime.

The first class was so well received that I scheduled another, then another. The written notes that I handed out kept getting more extensive. Soon, I realized that they needed to be accompanied by guided audio relaxation meditations. Then, the psychology department at my clinic asked to see what I'd created, so I put it all together for them. Eventually, as I taught and lectured more and more to groups and businesses about stress, the written materials evolved into a full book, especially for those people who were "too stressed to take a stress management course"!

The book and CD package you now hold in your hands is the final result of those 30 years of studying stress and 15 years of teaching people how to manage theirs. I've changed, refined, and, usually, simplified the techniques I teach over the years, after seeing what works and what doesn't.

I have tried to make the book neither gimmicky nor esoteric. When people are stressed, they don't have time for a 600-page tome. Therefore, this book is concise and to the point. I give you just the information you need to get proactive about stress relief as quickly as possible. If one of the topics strikes a chord with you, I encourage you to consult the reading list for more extensive study. I have included the points that people who have already taken my classes found most useful in dealing with stress, as well as a variety of pertinent quotations that add perspective and make for an entertaining and sometimes humorous read.

The first step in our journey will be to discover a technique that will help you effectively relax whenever you have a few free minutes. You can start using it right away while you learn more about stress in Chapter 2 and explore the in-depth relaxation techniques in Chapter 3. However, you don't always have a few free minutes. When your boss yells, "Get in here now!" it's best not to say, "I'll be there after my 10-minute relaxation break." If you did, you might end up with an extended relaxation break! Therefore, Chapters 4 and 5 explore a technique called *mindfulness* and show how it can be used to deal with stressful situations as they happen and can even alter their outcome. This deceptively simple technique is the heart of the book, and you may find, as I have, that its benefits go far beyond stress relief. In fact, it may help you discover greater happiness in every passing moment.

Closely connected to mindfulness, in Chapter 6, is the concept of changing your thoughts by reframing your mental context. Then, we will look at how slowing down can help with stress, and we will learn ways of putting our lives in perspective. Your physical health, and the amount you exercise, has a tremendous impact on stress levels, so we will investigate basic lifestyle changes that can minimize stress. Much stress revolves around relationships, so a discussion of communication skills is important. We will learn to deal with feelings of anger and frustration, take the stress out of decisions, and improve sleep.

Occasionally, even if you do all the right things to help yourself deal with stress, your surroundings are so stressful that internal solutions are insufficient. If your spouse regularly physically abuses you, exercise and meditation are going to get you only so far. Chapter 14 discusses when external changes are necessary and guides you in making those changes—but also cautions against the temptation to use your environment as an excuse. Chapter 15 teaches how best to combine all these strategies for maximum effect. Finally, in Chapter 16, I'll help you decide if your problems represent more than stress and, if so, what to do about it.

You will see that this book draws on a wide mixture of teachings, ranging from those of Albert Ellis and the Dalai Lama to those of Meyer Friedman and Jon Kabat-Zinn. Many of the techniques I created myself for my classes. The stories and anecdotes, which help illustrate concepts throughout the book, are drawn from my own life and from my patients and students. Their names and occupations have been changed to ensure their anonymity.

This is a hands-on book. It's here for your benefit. To get the most out of it, I encourage you to make it your own. Take notes in the book, underline meaningful parts, and consider the questions and exercises in each chapter. Instead of just reading the general techniques, actively tweak them so that they apply to your personal situation.

Throughout the book, you will find symbols marking four different types of activities for you to try:

⊙ Guided meditations using the enclosed CDs
❖ Nonguided exercises
🖉 Written questions or exercises (don't worry; no grading!)
⇨ Techniques to try in your daily work or home life

Even if you feel as if you already know some of these techniques, it is important to be reminded of the principles. I've taught well over a hundred stress management classes, yet every time I teach a class, I'm reminded of ways to handle my own stress more effectively. In the same way, if you are already familiar with some of the concepts presented in this book, *Take the Stress out of Your Life* should serve as an important reminder of common sense that is often forgotten.

In addition, you do not have to have severe problems with anxiety to benefit from *Take the Stress out of Your Life*. Just because you aren't suffering from psoriasis or high blood pressure doesn't mean stress isn't sapping some of the pleasure from your life. Even people with low levels of stress find that the skills taught in this book improve their day-to-day lives. In fact, you can think of them as basic training for a rewarding and productive life. After all, learning to fully experience every moment is something from which we can all benefit. You would not expect to run a marathon without training your body. You would not expect to work at almost any professional occupation without instruction. In order to live the most joyful life possible, you must have some basic instruction and must train your mind. My students have ranged from people with minimal stress to people with full-blown anxiety disorders. Virtually all of them came away with useful information.

There is no ultimate, quick fix for stress. Learning to manage it well is a lifelong pursuit. However, completing this book and trying the exercises in it and on the CD set will be a very healthy start to the endeavor.

Congratulate yourself for starting the journey to a healthier and happier life. If you make the commitment to finish the book and follow through with the recommendations, your life may never be the same.

SOME STRESSFUL FACTS

○ One million U.S. employees miss work every day because of stress.
○ Research has shown stress to be the number one impediment to academic success.
○ Work-related stress doubles the risk of dying from heart disease and stroke.
○ A study showed that individuals who did stress management training had 74 percent less recurrent heart disease than those who did not have the training.
○ People with high levels of stress had about twice the risk of Alzheimer's disease.
○ Health care expenses are nearly 50 percent greater for workers under high levels of stress.

🖉 Goals Exercise

What benefits would you like from completing this book and CD set? Check all that apply, and feel free to add more:

❑   Decreased feelings of anxiety

❑   Decreased worry

❑   Improved productivity at work and/or school

❑   Improved relationships at work

❑   Improved relationships at home

❑   Improved sleep

❑   Improved health

❑   More joy

❑   Improvement in specific medical problems and/or symptoms. Please list:

Take the Stress out of Your Life

1

Quick-Start: Reduce Your Stress in Six Minutes

SOME PEOPLE ARE suspicious of meditation, perhaps because of the New Age trappings that sometimes clothe it. Or they are skeptical that a few minutes of sitting could have any impact on their physical state. Those people are usually quite surprised when they take my course and find themselves significantly more relaxed after a single meditation. If you have any skepticism toward meditation, or think you won't be able to successfully do it, the following exercise, which takes just six minutes, will show you that meditation is (A) incredibly simple and (B) incredibly effective.

At some point in your day, when you have ten free minutes and access to a computer or CD player, take a moment to rank your current stress level:

0___1___2___3___4___5___6___7___8___9___10

Extremely relaxed   Extremely tense

⊙ Six-Minute Meditation. Disk 1, Track 1. Length: Six Minutes

Without trying too hard to relax, play the assigned track and follow the instructions. There are no requirements, though you'll probably want to choose a spot with few distractions and a comfortable place to sit.

Now rank how you feel:

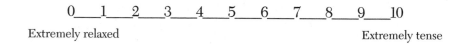

0___1___2___3___4___5___6___7___8___9___10
Extremely relaxed   Extremely tense

While you may not feel wildly transformed by that exercise, you probably found yourself more relaxed, focused, and content when the meditation was over. You managed your stress. In six minutes! As we get deeper into the book, the meditations and other techniques will get more in-depth, but if you were able to do that exercise, you'll have no problem with the rest.

2

Good Stress/Bad Stress

The process of living is the process of reacting to stress.
STANLEY J. SARNOFF

IF I ASKED YOU if you wanted stress, your response would likely be "Are you crazy?" Most people think stress is as useless as an air conditioner in an igloo. But tell that to the caveman who narrowly escaped the jaws of a saber-toothed tiger. That boost of adrenaline helped him avoid being the special entrée of the day.

But surely today things are different. Nowadays, we need stress like we need dinosaur-hunting gear, right? The truth is that stress is as much a part of us as is our brain or heart. When the system is working right, it can help us accomplish important things. One night I was sound asleep when I was awakened by the sound of my five-year-old son screaming. I did not get out of bed in the usual fashion. From a sound sleep, I vaulted over my wife and made it down a flight of stairs and to my son's side in less than five seconds. When I got there, I discovered that the emergency was that his covers had fallen off, but the point is that I could not normally have accomplished that vault, stair descent, and run in five seconds. With the help of an adrenaline

5

burst, I was able to do it from a sound sleep. And if there had been a real emergency, those precious seconds could have made all the difference.

If you are tired and are either taking an exam or playing in a tennis match, a little extra adrenaline can actually improve your performance. But indeed, as we all know, there can be too much of a good thing. Too much adrenaline spells "F" on your exam and isn't so great for your tennis game, either.

In short, a certain amount of stress can be helpful. We call this good stress *eustress*. The extra energy or adrenaline is often felt as excitement, passion, and enthusiasm. When we go over our stress quota, however, we enter the land of *distress*. That's often felt as anxiety, worry, and a tight knot in your stomach. Other signs of distress are muscular tension, fatigue, racing heart, insomnia, irritability, shakiness, excessive sweating, upset stomach, lack of appetite, and a sense of being overwhelmed.

Excessive and prolonged distress can lead to the myriad of health, relationship, and work performance problems discussed in the introduction. And, of course, it feels miserable. With high levels of prolonged stress, not only is too much adrenaline released, but excessive amounts of the hormone cortisol are also spewed from your adrenal glands. Cortisol can decrease inflammation, but it also has some less desirable effects. It decreases your immunity and makes it harder to fight off infections. It makes you ravenous (supposedly to make up for the calories you burned in "fight or flight") and encourages storage of the new calories as belly fat—the very type of fat that is associated with diabetes, heart disease, and stroke. To complicate matters further, if adrenaline has your motor running way over the recommended RPMs for a long time, you're on the expressway to the junk heap. It's time for an overhaul before it's too late!

So how might we start in our quest not only to manage stress, but also to thrive under the stressful conditions commonplace in the 21st century? Stress management techniques can be grouped into two broad categories: external changes we can make in our lives, and internal changes we can make by modifying our thought processes. Often, a combination of both external and internal changes is the best remedy in our manic world.

Sometimes the need to make external change is obvious. If you have a size 9 foot, but are wearing size 6 shoes and your feet hurt, don't just sit there and try to bear it; get new shoes! If your spouse beats you, it may be best to find a shelter and move out, because no amount of internal changing is going to remedy the situation. If there is a better job down the street, perhaps you should quit your current one. Toward the end of the book, we'll look at making important external changes.

However, don't fool yourself into believing that the problem is always external, or that one more change of environment will solve everything. If you expect to find a job that lives perfectly up to all your desires, you'd better start exploring a new planet, because it's not happening on Earth! If you want to find the relationship in which you are always treated exactly how you think you should be treated, it's a new galaxy you'll need to find! Far more often, the source of bad stress is not the external world itself but our way of dealing with it. That's fortunate, because it means that with this book and a little introspection, you have everything you need to manage your stress.

Even minor changes in your internal response can dramatically influence the way you deal with stress. Some people, such as brain surgeons and police officers, flourish in what others would consider very stressful jobs, while others experience overwhelming amounts of distress in seemingly relaxed jobs. In the following chapters, we'll unravel the puzzle of why this is so, and you'll master the skills needed to thrive in this stressful world. Let's start by learning to relax.

The last of the human freedoms—to choose one's attitude in any given set of circumstances, to choose one's own way.

VICTOR FRANKL

3

Learn to Relax

Relaxing is like playing an instrument. To become proficient we must practice, practice, practice.

PIERRE

You don't start learning to be a brain surgeon by cutting into someone's brain. It always pays to start with the basics. Likewise, the first step in staying relaxed throughout the day is learning to relax for a specified period of time. Let's start by learning to relax for 10 minutes. This is no easy task for many. If you've ever tried to relax during some free time but found that you couldn't unwind, or if you've found that when bedtime arrived relaxation was out of reach, then you know what I'm talking about. Wouldn't it be nice to be able to fully relax and unwind whenever you had a few free minutes? But even that's not the best part! Once you learn this skill, it will lay the foundation for being able to relax and enjoy your whole day regardless of free time. In Chapters 4 and 5, you will expand your skills to be able to enjoy life in the midst of your busiest day.

Just as your body can have a stress response, it can also have a relaxation response, which clears stress hormones from the blood, slows your heart rate, and softens your hyperalertness. A sense of calm and well-being returns. It's this response—and the health benefits it provides—that we're after when we train ourselves to relax.

9

There are multiple relaxation exercises, but I'm not going to waste your time with an endless catalog of these techniques. Remember, my job is not only to present a technique that will relax you for the moment but also to teach important skills that can be applied to the rest of the day. In that light, we will learn a simple and versatile type of meditation.

If you have any preconceived ideas about meditation, please put them aside. Although every religion teaches some style of meditation, meditation in itself is not religious. It is not New Age—in fact, it's been around for thousands of years. It is a basic skill that should be taught in kindergarten. (If you already know how to meditate, don't miss this important review.) By learning this technique, you will learn skills that can be applied during a normal day—making your days much less stressful and more enjoyable.

Meditation has been shown to decrease stress and increase feelings of well-being. A variety of health benefits have also been associated with meditation, including improvement in headaches, high blood pressure, psoriasis, and chronic pain. Over the course of approximately 19 years of study of people with high blood pressure, people who meditated had a 23 percent decreased chance of dying. Additionally, regular meditation seems to increase activity in an area of the brain associated with happiness and well-being called the *left prefrontal cortex*. A recent study found that long-term meditators actually had important structural changes in the brain. As people age, the cortex, the outer part of the brain, thins. Long-term meditators had cortices that remained thicker than those in the people who did not meditate.

Sarah was experiencing leg cramps one evening and decided to listen to the meditation on Track 2 of the first CD. By the time the meditation was over, her leg pain was gone.

Similarly, Bob was having a headache when he started listening to the CD. His headache was 50 percent better by the end of the meditation.

Beth was 78 years old and was very concerned about how she would tolerate a one-hour dental procedure. She decided that the dental chair would be an ideal spot to practice her meditation. Before she knew it, the procedure was over and the dentist was amazed at how well Beth had done.

Amy was a 39-year-old physical therapist when she first saw me. Her blood pressure was very elevated and she was having trouble coping with her work-related stress. I told her that her treatment would likely include blood pressure medication, but first, I recommended that she address her diet, exercise, and stress management. She started meditating daily and working on the mindfulness techniques described in the next chapter. When I saw her at our next visit two weeks later, her blood pressure was normal without medication, and she was coping with work much better.*

The first step I usually recommend in learning meditation is diaphragmatic breathing. The diaphragm is a large dome-shaped muscle that separates the chest from the abdomen. As you breathe in, the diaphragm contracts and flattens out. The lungs fill the lower chest cavity and the abdomen expands (see Figure 1). When people are anxious, they tend to breathe without using the

---

*Note of caution: It is very important to get regular screenings for high blood pressure and not to stop blood pressure medication without a doctor's supervision. Untreated high blood pressure is associated with a significantly high risk of stroke and heart attack. Although some studies have shown a reduction of blood pressure from regular meditation, many people still require medication.

diaphragm and, instead, use the muscles in the neck and chest. They also tend to breathe quickly or to hyperventilate. Among other effects, hyperventilation temporarily alters the acid-base balance of the blood, increasing feelings of anxiety.

Diaphragmatic breathing is both an important component of meditation and a relaxation exercise in its own right. One of the benefits of diaphragmatic breathing is that it is much more relaxing. Breathing with your diaphragm activates the *parasympathetic nervous system*—the part of your nervous system that is in charge of the relaxation response. Sometimes a few nice, deep breaths are all you need to be calmer.

❖ Diaphragmatic Breathing

Breathe in through your nose, and let your abdomen gently move outward with each inhalation. As you initially learn diaphragmatic breathing, it may be helpful to put one hand on your abdomen. Let your hand rise with each breath in. You may breathe out through your nose or mouth. If you have trouble getting comfortable with this style of breathing, try breathing while lying flat on your back.

If you are still having trouble getting the hang of diaphragmatic breathing, don't get frustrated. Be patient and give yourself time to get used to it. When I was in college, an exercise physiologist performed free posture evaluations as part of a research study. I was advised to stand with my shoulders further back. Initially, this position seemed very strange and awkward. However, within a few weeks, my improved posture felt natural. Similarly, as you practice the diaphragmatic breathing, it will become more natural.

Tom was a busy corporate executive who came to me complaining of coughing fits that had been going on for over a month. He

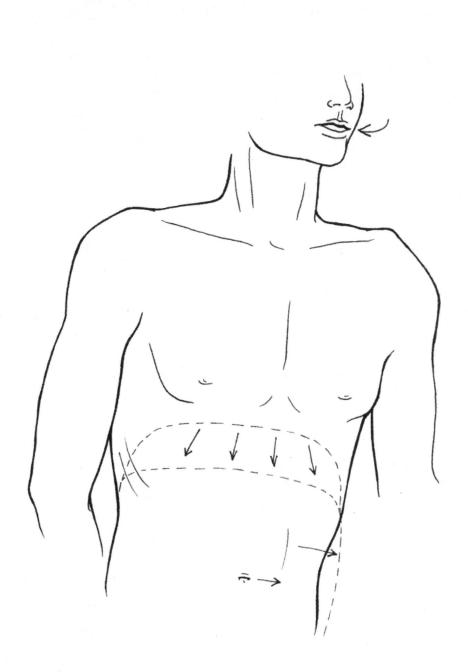

FIGURE 1
With each breath in, the diaphragm contracts and flattens,
forcing the abdomen out.

would have four or five of the fits per day. The fits would start as a tickle in his throat; then he would start coughing and feel as if he could not get a full breath. When he was in an important business meeting, he would start to worry about having a coughing fit, and invariably he would start coughing. A previous doctor had prescribed antibiotics, but the fits persisted.

As we were discussing the various options to treat his problem, Tom started getting a "tickle" in his throat. However, this time, with my guidance, he focused on slow, diaphragmatic breaths, and he didn't get the coughing fit that usually followed. Tom ended up not needing the prescription medicine we had considered trying.

Jim was in his 50s and had a long history of Parkinson's disease. To add to his challenges, he had developed heart disease and, later, a rare tumor of his stomach called a carcinoid. He required a major surgery to remove the tumor and part of his stomach.

As he was coming out of the anesthesia, he realized that he had missed his Parkinson's disease medication. His body felt stiff and he was losing control of his muscles. He became very anxious. His heart raced and he started to feel short of breath. Then he remembered what he had learned in my stress management class. Although he was uncomfortable, he focused on diaphragmatic breathing, and his heart rate dropped. Soon he was no longer short of breath and he started feeling much better.

Once you learn diaphragmatic breathing, you are ready to move on and learn meditation. It is best to be comfortable as you practice meditation.

Begin your meditation when you are not excessively hungry, thirsty, or full. Try to wear loose, comfortable clothing that does not constrict your chest or waist, and find a comfortable place to sit down. Meditation may be done while sitting up straight in a chair with your arms and legs uncrossed, while sitting on a pillow on the floor, or while lying down. On Track 2 of the first CD, I will guide you in learning to meditate. I will ask you to focus primarily on your breath as it flows in and out. As you listen, remember to use diaphragmatic breathing.

As you meditate, you will probably have many thoughts. This is normal. As a thought comes into your mind, simply notice it and then let it go—return your focus to your breath. By mastering the ability to observe your thoughts in a nonjudgmental fashion and let them go, you will be well on your way to coping effectively with many stressful situations.*

⊙ Relaxation Meditation. Disk 1, Track 2. Length: 20 Minutes

Find somewhere quiet, choose a comfortable position, and listen to the CD. There are approximately 16 minutes of guided meditation, followed by 4 minutes of silence, occasionally interrupted by the sound of a bell. The bells serve two purposes. An individual bell reminds you to return to noticing your breath. A series of three bells alerts you that you have been meditating for 20 minutes. If you are pressed for time, you can do the 16 minutes of meditation and skip the 4 minutes of silence. If you are *really* pressed for time, you should do the 6-minute meditation on Disk 1, Track 1, instead (especially if you didn't do it earlier). Never listen to the CD while driving or while operating potentially dangerous machinery.

---

*During the guided meditation, you will be asked to avoid resisting body sensations. Although serious medical problems (such as heart problems) are less likely during relaxation, they can occur at any time. Therefore, never ignore any severe pain, chest pain, or significant breathing problems.

These meditations may be used repeatedly. After a few sessions, you may decide to meditate without the CD.

Reading about meditation may seem a little dry. However, by the end of Chapter 4, you will see how meditation provides a foundation for learning to deal with stress throughout the day.

16 Tips for Good Meditation

1. **View your** meditation sessions as a reward, as time you set aside for yourself, not as another chore or task to complete.

2. **When you** learn to meditate, it is ideal to be in a comfortable setting. It is best to learn in quiet surroundings. Later, you may enjoy the challenge of a noisier setting. You can let any noise be a signal for you to go deeper into your meditation. You may need to be creative in finding times to meditate. For many, first thing in the morning is easiest. After I read their bedtime stories, my children enjoy my sitting on their bed and meditating as they fall asleep.

3. **Positions suitable** for meditation include: sitting in a chair with your legs uncrossed and your hands flat on your lap, sitting on a pillow on the floor, or lying on your back. One disadvantage—or perhaps, advantage—of meditating lying down is that you may fall asleep during the meditation. Falling asleep may be an advantage if it is time to go to bed, but a disadvantage on a workday morning. If you are sitting as you meditate, assume a dignified posture with your back straight.

4. **Start with** diaphragmatic breathing, and focus on the sensation of breathing in your nostrils, throat, lungs, and/or abdomen. You can pick the spot easiest to notice. Many find it most relaxing to focus on the abdomen. Pay attention to the full duration of the in breath and the full duration of the out breath. The idea is to focus on and enjoy the sensation of

just this breath. To give a sense of enjoying the sensation of breathing, people have used descriptions such as "tasting the breath" or even "luxuriating in the breath." If you find that the diaphragmatic breathing is too difficult or uncomfortable, then just watch your breath as it is. Some meditation traditions recommend that you not manipulate your breath, the object being just to feel the breath as it is. As you become more relaxed, you may find you are naturally breathing using your diaphragm.

5. **When thoughts** come to mind, do not resist them. Instead of judging the thoughts, just notice them, and then gently let them go. You might imagine each thought as a cloud floating by, or a branch floating down a stream. Do not be discouraged if you have an abundance of thoughts. Meditation is not about having zero thoughts, but about developing your ability to gently let the thoughts go as soon as they appear. After letting each thought go, pay full attention to, and enjoy, your very next breath. Each thought you have provides you more practice in the skill of quickly letting thoughts go. Don't be surprised if your meditation sessions initially consist of a lot of thinking and only a few minutes focused on the breath. A transcript of your thoughts during a meditation might read: " . . . I have a bunch of dishes to do. I also need to get a lot of work done tomorrow—oh yeah, I'm meditating. . . . I wonder what time . . . My back . . ." Don't worry; as long as you learn to gently let the thoughts go and focus on your next breath, the meditation is working.

6. **Although I** described meditation as a way to relax, it is best not to try too hard to relax. It is enough to just listen to the CDs and follow the instructions in this chapter. Ironically, if you do try too hard to relax, relaxation may elude you. If you are meditating by focusing on your breath, just focus on your

breath and nonjudgmentally observe your physical sensations and thoughts. If you have 1,000 distracting thoughts, just gently bring your attention back 1,001 times. You can be thankful for that moment when you "wake up" and realize your attention has drifted.

7. **Avoid resisting** your body sensations. Sometimes the more you resist an uncomfortable sensation, the more spasm you create in the surrounding area. When you stop resisting the sensation, sometimes the discomfort eases.

8. **You might** try a body scan toward the beginning of the meditation. Relax one part of your body at a time, starting either with your feet or with your head and working your way along your entire body.

9. **Another alternative** to focusing on your breath is to focus on a repetitive phrase, called a mantra. Thich Nhat Hahn, a renowned meditation teacher, suggests repeating the following statements to yourself: "Breathing in, I calm my body; breathing out, I smile," and with the next breath, "Dwelling in the present moment" (as you inhale), "I know this is a wonderful moment" (as you exhale). To shorten the phrases you can try "calm—smile; present moment—wonderful moment." Hahn also recommends meditating with a half smile on your face. Herbert Benson, M.D., a prominent mind-body researcher, believes that people with a religious tradition may gain additional benefit from repeating a short prayer as a mantra. He believes that repetition of the short prayer phrase lets the mind and body remember additional feelings of wellness. Other potential mantras include: "one," "love," "peace," "relax," or any other word or phrase that you find relaxing and/or meaningful. You may experiment to find the phrase or phrases that work best for you. Have you ever had a song run through your mind long after you heard it?

In the same way, a meaningful mantra may linger with you throughout the day.

10. **Generally, it** is best to continue the meditation session uninterrupted. If you occasionally have very important thoughts, you can keep a notepad and pencil by you. If you decide to do this, however, you should use the notepad rarely. The notepad becomes useful if otherwise you would be spending 20 minutes worried about forgetting, or actually forgetting, an important responsibility (such as picking someone up at the airport).

11. **I recommend** starting your meditation practice with your eyes closed. Later, you can try meditating with your eyes open. When your eyes are open, you can maintain an unfocused gaze or focus on an object, such as a flower or a candle.

12. **If you'd** like, you may end the meditation with a phrase, such as giving thanks for the present moment, the people in your life, your health, and so on.

13. **Like exercise**, you can use meditation as you need it. However, there is much benefit to incorporating meditation into your daily routine. Perhaps, instead of hitting the snooze button several times, you might sit up in bed, when the alarm goes off, and do a meditation to start your day. Alternatively, right after work or before dinner may be a good time for you.

14. **There are** different opinions about how long to meditate. For instance, when people begin learning Transcendental Meditation, or TM, they are usually asked to meditate for 20 minutes, twice a day. At the University of Massachusetts Mindfulness-Based Stress Reduction program, it is recommended that people meditate (or do a similar exercise) for 40 minutes a day. There is no perfect amount of time to meditate. In fact, an interesting study would be to see how people benefit from different meditation schedules. I suggest that you meditate at least 10 minutes a day and, on

occasion, meditate at least a few minutes after you have the thought, "I feel like stopping." It is nice to realize that you do not have to respond to a thought as soon as you have it and, instead, can enjoy a few more minutes of meditation.

15. **If you** want to try to meditate without the CDs, consider using a timer so you know when the meditation is over. That way you do not have to keep checking your watch. Any timer will do, but there are a variety of timers explicitly for meditation. These timers tend to have a pleasant bell or chime to signify the end of the period. There are free online meditation timers, CDs used to time meditation, and stand-alone timers that can be purchased.

16. **Like many** things, meditation takes practice and dedication. Just as it takes time to build your muscles with physical exercise, your ability to focus will improve as you exercise it with meditation. Do not expect one meditation session to be like another. It is helpful to continue your regular practice despite any thoughts of boredom or discontent. There is a great deal to be learned from meditating when your mind is distracted. Learning to deal with distracting thoughts in meditation will teach you important skills that can be used throughout the day. Buddhist nun and author Pema Chödrön stated, "I've had many times when I meditate, and it seems like my mind is just going a hundred miles an hour. And yet, when I stand up and walk into life, there's more room in my mind."

When does meditation fit into your day?_____

_____

4

Learn to Enjoy Your Day

In order to be utterly happy, the only thing necessary is to refrain from comparing this moment with other moments in the past, which I often did not fully enjoy because I was comparing them with other moments of the future.

ANDRI GIDE

ENJOYABLE, HEALTHY ACTIVITIES, such as hiking, bathing, eating, watching a sunset, and listening to music, are good for you and can reduce your stress level. However, if you obsess about your problems as you participate in these activities, the benefit will be minimal. Eating a healthy gourmet meal can help reduce stress, but only if you taste the food, rather than spend the time worrying about problems at work. Playing tennis can be a relaxing activity, but not if you spend most of the game angry at yourself for not playing well.

The purpose of this chapter is to help you make your relaxing activities truly relaxing and your stressful activities less stressful and more enjoyable. An extremely effective method of doing this is the practice of mindfulness. Mindfulness has evolved over thousands of years, and because of its effectiveness, it is a cornerstone of this book.

The Present Moment

Simply put, mindfulness involves nonjudgmentally focusing your attention on the present moment. To begin exploring the concept of mindfulness, consider this question: "How many ways can the present be—not tomorrow, not five minutes from now, not even one second from now, but this very moment?" The present moment can be only one way. In other words, the present moment can be only as it is. In five seconds we may be able to effect a change, but right now can exist only the way it is.

Nevertheless, the average person spends a tremendous amount of time wishing that the present moment were different. As soon as the alarm goes off in the morning, a stream of thoughts begins: "I don't feel like waking up now. . . . I wish I didn't have to go to work. . . . If only it weren't so cold and rainy out. . . . I wish the kids would be quieter. . . . If only my spouse/boss/friend would act differently. . . . I wish my back felt better. . . . I feel overwhelmed" and so on. What a stressful way to begin the day! It is a useful exercise to start paying attention to how much time during your day you spend wishing that the present moment was different.

Applying Mindfulness

By applying the mindfulness skills learned in meditation, you can turn a potentially aggravating situation into a more pleasant experience. For instance, let's say you are stressed while in a traffic jam. When you think about it, a traffic jam should be a low-stress experience. There are not a lot of decisions to make. All we usually need to do is follow the car in front of us. A trained monkey could almost do that! Why is it stressful? Most likely, we are saying or thinking something to the effect of "I wish I weren't here. . . . What bad luck I have. . . . Those other drivers are idiots.

. . . I can't be late. . . ." In other words, we wish the present moment were different.

Instead of spending the next 30 minutes stressed out, take what you learned in your meditation and use it. Don't get angry at the negative thoughts; they are a normal response. When you notice the thoughts, gently let them go and notice your next breath. Perhaps those thoughts will come up again and again. Each time a thought arises, you can gently let it go in the same nonjudgmental fashion. Don't worry if a particular negative thought occurs frequently. The skill lies in seeing how quickly you can let the thought go, so that you can enjoy the present moment just as it is. As in the meditation practice, each thought gives you an additional opportunity to practice the skill of letting thoughts go gently and quickly. If a thought comes up 100 times, great—you've got 100 times to practice.

Importance of Thoughts and Goals

Mindfulness practice is not meant to discourage thought. Without our thoughts, we would not know how to tie our shoes, much less use a computer or cure life-threatening diseases. However, a key to managing stress and enjoying life is learning how to let certain nonproductive thoughts go, enabling ourselves to enjoy the present moment.

Practicing mindfulness does not mean our goals should be abandoned. Without goals, we would accomplish very little. There are times when it is appropriate to think about the future and to make plans. When we are mindful, we learn from our past and plan our future, but by not obsessing on either; we do not lose sight of the present moment.

We can and should work to make changes in the future, but in doing so, we should also challenge ourselves to enjoy the process. Reinhold Niebuhr wrote, in the often-quoted serenity prayer,

"God give me the serenity to accept things which cannot be changed; Give me courage to change things which must be changed; And the wisdom to distinguish one from the other. " I would add, "Please give us the understanding that change often takes time and the wisdom to enjoy the process of change." In other words, we should use mindfulness as a tool to enjoy the journey. Without mindfulness, life can become a never-ending series of desires, with little enjoyment of the here and now. While in high school, we can't wait to graduate and enter college. As college students, we want to graduate and start working. When working, we might wish for retirement. Maybe we think that life will be better if we are married; or if we're married, we think that divorce will bring us happiness. If happiness were achieved only when our goals are met, our happiness would be short-lived indeed, since another "goal" is always around the corner.

For a long time it had seemed to me that life was about to begin—real life. But there was always some obstacle in the way, something to be got through first, some unfinished business, time still to be served, a debt to be paid. Then life would begin. At last it dawned on me that these obstacles were my life.

ALFRED D' SOUZA

Mindfulness and Stress

Even a small increase in the amount of mindfulness can dramatically improve the way that you handle stress in your life. Figure 2 illustrates an escalating stress problem. As successive stressful events occur, they act cumulatively and result in an elevated level of stress. When this high level of stress is sustained for long periods of time, both physical and emotional problems are likely to arise. In contrast, each time you bring yourself to enjoy the present moment, even for

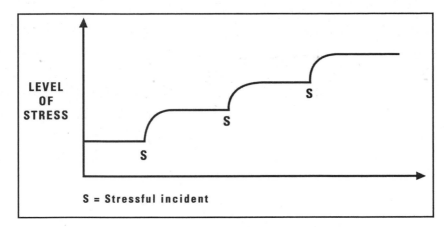

FIGURE 2
Stress is more harmful when it continues to rise and stays elevated.

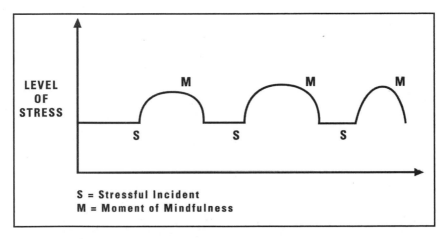

FIGURE 3
As you can see, even a few episodes of mindfulness make
a significant difference in how you handle stress.

a short period of time, you decrease your level of stress (see Figure 3). Every moment you are mindful not only brings more relaxation to that moment but also decreases the stress in the moments that follow. As Figure 3 demonstrates, with just a few moments of mindfulness the stress fails to reach the high level in Figure 2. It is unrealistic to expect that you will be mindful 100 percent of the time. However, an increase in mindfulness from 1 percent to just 2 percent of the time doubles your stress reduction.

The Stress Cycle

Sometimes people elevate their anxiety level by trying to resist their anxious feelings. In other words, they get anxious about being anxious—stressed about being stressed. Figure 4 illustrates this type of nonproductive cycle.

If your heart is pounding fast and you don't like the feeling, you might resist the sensation and wish your heart would slow down (Figure 4, Arrow 1). "I hate how I feel. I hope my heart slows

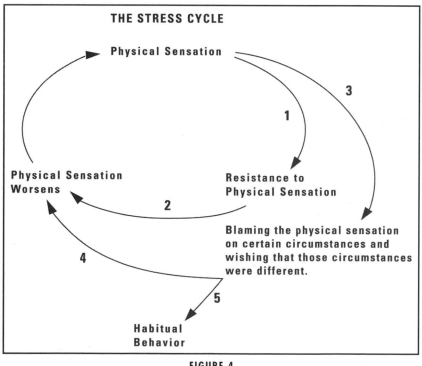

FIGURE 4
The Stress Cycle

down! It's going way too fast." Guess what happens next? That's right—your heart goes faster than a supersonic jet! The more you resist the sensation, the faster your heart pounds and the worse you feel (Figure 4, Arrow 2). In addition to this cycle, another cycle may contribute to the anxiety. For instance, you might blame the anxiety on your supervisor's actions. If you focus your thoughts on wishing that your boss behaved differently, you end up resisting the present circumstance (Figure 4, Arrow 3). Your heart rate and anxiety then further increase (Figure 4, Arrow 4).

Some people attempt to relieve stress by engaging in an automatic behavior or habit, such as smoking, nail-biting, or overeating (Figure 4, Arrow 5). These habits are largely nonproductive and may be harmful in the long run. Of course, for the most part, people are not consciously choosing deleterious behavior. Their bodies react in a way that they've unconsciously learned may give them temporary relief—even if it exacerbates the problem in the long run. However, the temporary relief is still relief, and it's the best solution they can come up with at the time.

But we can do better! Let's look at another way of handling the situation. When a patient comes to me complaining of a racing heart, I start by asking enough questions to reassure both of us that the sensation is not caused by a medical problem.* If the racing heart is caused by anxiety, as it most frequently is, I tell my patient to let his or her heart beat as fast as it can. That's right—I instruct the person to sit down, take some diaphragmatic breaths, and let his or her heart beat as fast as it likes. This technique often slows the racing heart and decreases the anxiety because it breaks the vicious circle described in Figure 4. The person is no longer resisting the physical sensation.

---

*See Chapter 16, page 212, for information on evaluating palpitations (the sensation of a prominent, fast, or irregular heartbeat).

Similarly, making a conscious effort not to resist external circumstances, such as your supervisor's behavior, can also decrease your stress level. Perhaps you can change his or her future behavior with some tactful feedback. However, for the present moment, focusing on the wish that your boss were different is counterproductive.

If you notice yourself engaging in an automatic behavior or habit, pay attention to the physical sensations and thoughts that tend to occur before that behavior. Let the associated thoughts go as you focus on your breath. Rather than "running away" from the uncomfortable physical sensations by grabbing a cigarette or habitually turning on the television, try to sit with the feeling for a few moments. By accepting the knot in your stomach, and taking some mindful diaphragmatic breaths, you may find that the discomfort decreases or passes altogether. By resisting a sensation, we often make it worse than it would otherwise be.

It is ideal to break the cycle described in Figure 4 as soon as it starts. Don't spend 20 minutes wishing things were different. As soon as you notice a "resistant thought," let the thought go, and focus on your next breath. As with meditation, if the thought comes up again, patiently let it go again. Remember that the more thoughts you have, the more practice you gain in letting the thoughts go. Be patient with yourself. Each time you realize that your mind has drifted, be thankful for that realization and bring your attention back to the present. Also, as with meditation, remember to breathe using your diaphragm. By learning to recognize the thoughts and feelings of stress early, you can break the stress cycle before it starts, or at least before it goes very far.

Pay attention to your body. Do you tend to tense certain muscle groups when under stress? Typical muscle groups that tense in the stress response include those in the neck, shoulders, back, abdomen, hands, jaw, and face (especially the little muscles between the eyes). If you typically tense your shoulders as you get stressed, learn to focus on your shoulders as soon as you notice the stress. As you focus on your shoulders, allow them to relax just as you did during the first two meditations on Disk 1. The muscle relaxation is easiest when you do it early in the stress response.

✏ Tense-Muscle Identification

Take a moment to list the muscle groups that tend to tense the most when you are stressed. If you don't know the answer now, pay attention to your body when you are next stressed, and then fill in the list.

1. _____

2. _____

3. _____

4. _____

In summary, when you find yourself stressed and wishing the present moment were different, simply let the thought go, focus on a diaphragmatic breath or other present-moment sensation (such as hearing, sight, taste, and touch), and perhaps relax a muscle group. If you like, you can focus on the abdomen expanding with the in breath, and focus on a muscle group relaxing with the out breath.

Sam was 17 years old when he came to see me. He was having recurrent headaches and nausea. He hated taking medications and wanted to explore other treatment options. Sam experienced stress about several different issues in his life, such as his high school basketball games. Typically, he would feel a little nervous, wish he felt different, and start clenching his jaw. Soon his headache would begin. After we talked, Sam tried another approach. As soon as he felt himself starting to get stressed or wishing he felt different, he would let the thoughts go, focus on diaphragmatic breathing, and relax his jaw. By the time of our next visit, Sam's headaches were occurring much less frequently.

Eustress

Adopting the right attitude can convert a negative stress into a positive one.

HANS SELYE

Many people like roller coasters, but not all enjoy the beginning of the ride. Your palms get sweaty, your heart pounds, and your pupils dilate. You quietly (or not so quietly) cuss out the friend who talked you into taking this stupid ride. When you reach the top of the roller coaster and look down that first big hill, you're convinced you're going to die! As the ride continues, you find yourself excited and enjoying the swift turns. Wait a minute— what happened? Your heart is still pounding fast, your palms are still sweaty, and your pupils are still dilated, but now you're having fun. What's different?

At the beginning of the ride, maybe you wished that you were somewhere else and that your body wasn't so tense. But by the middle and end of the ride, you just accepted the ride for what it was and enjoyed the rush. In other words, as you stopped resisting the experience, the anxiety was transformed into excitement.

In Chapter 2, I discussed how not all stress is bad. There is bad stress, called *distress*, and good stress, called *eustress*. Now say the word *eustress* slowly out loud. *Eustress* sounds a lot like *use stress*, doesn't it? And that's a good way to think of it. How many performers have gotten up in front of thousands of people and never had a surge of adrenaline? Probably not many. The good ones learn to use that excess energy. At times, it is best to handle stress by using the additional energy to be excited and to enthusiastically pursue your goals.

Although not all stress is bad, the statement "I'm stressed" has a very negative connotation to most people. Just the thought of being stressed can lead us to resist our feelings. In turn, the more we resist stress, the more distressed we get. In a sense, we get anxious about being anxious. Solution? One strategy is to replace the thoughts "I'm stressed" or "I'm stressed out" with the thoughts "I have a high energy level" or "My adrenaline level is up" and then to use the energy. Even if you don't actively "use" the energy, you can, in a sense, welcome it. Let go of the thoughts of how you should feel different and fully embrace the sensations just as they are. By reframing the situation in this way, you can let yourself enjoy how your body feels in the moment, as opposed to resisting the sensations. Sometimes you might lessen stress by listening to mellow music. Other times, you might manage stress by singing and dancing to an upbeat tune.

❖ The Use-Stress Challenge

1. **When you** feel stressed and you are in an appropriate setting, see how it feels to say to yourself, "Great! I have a high energy level." Let go of any thoughts to the contrary. Assume the attitude of being thankful for the extra energy. Then turn on some music and dance, or go out for a run with some upbeat music on your MP3 player. You will likely find this activity works to convert the distress to eustress.
2. **The next** time you feel stressed, try again saying to yourself, "Great! I have a high energy level." Feel the desired energy course through your veins. This time, do [or] continue your normal activity with this extra energy.

Enjoying the Present

The purpose of life is to live it, to taste experience to the utmost, to reach out eagerly and without fear for richer and newer experience.

ELEANOR ROOSEVELT

To further explore mindfulness, consider how your mind works when you are feeling your best. Take a moment to recall a peak experience, such as gazing into your lover's eyes, holding your newborn child, walking on the beach during a sunset, standing on a surfboard for the first time, or skiing in deep powder. Let's pretend your peak experience was watching a beach sunset. During the peak experience, I know you weren't thinking, "It's OK, but I wish there was a little less pink and a little more orange." Instead, you simply savored the magic as the sunset unfolded. Perhaps you thought that particular beach was great for sunsets, so you later went back to it. However, the next time, you found yourself not just enjoying the sunset, but comparing it to the previous sunset. And guess what. No peak experience. It wasn't that particular beach that caused the peak experience. It was how you were— how you mindfully enjoyed the moment. All peak experiences have a common element. They occur when you are fully present, enjoying the moment just as it is, as opposed to wishing this or that were different.

The mindfulness that spontaneously helps us appreciate a peak experience can also help us find joy in simple activities. Taking a shower, eating, driving, walking, or even doing the dishes can become a relaxation exercise. When we wash dishes, we are often thinking about how we would like to be done already. Instead, Thich Nhat Hanh does a dishwashing meditation: He fills the sink and enjoys the feeling of his hands in the warm sudsy water— enjoying washing one dish at a time.

The opportunities to enjoy the present moment are limitless. We can enjoy the next breath, the next step, the warm water in the shower, the cold water in the pool, or the many different aromas from the smell of dinner to the smell of a flower. Instead of being totally distracted when we eat or comparing our current meal to another, we can take a few seconds to smell the aroma, to look at the food, and to notice the texture and how it feels in different parts of our mouths.

During one session of my stress management class, we do a meditation in which we very slowly savor one strawberry for about 10 minutes. We appreciate the unique appearance of the strawberry and enjoy its fragrance, texture, and taste. A classic type of meditation is the walking meditation. Next time you walk from one office to the next, instead of worrying about your work, notice each breath and notice the ground massaging your feet with every step. You can also enjoy the input from your eyes. As you notice each breath and let your thoughts go, you'll start noticing that what at first appeared to be boring, everyday scenery is actually worthy of a postcard.

Turn everyday routines into special moments of relaxation. Make a bath or shower into a meditation: Feel the warm water on your body, enjoy your fingers massaging your scalp as you shampoo, notice the soap lather, and feel the texture of the towel as you dry off. Even as you brush your teeth, you can notice the bristles of the brush massaging your gums. As you pet your dog or cat, pay attention to how the fur feels on your fingers and hands. Notice the scenery to enjoy your trip to work. Do some mindful stretching (on your own or in a yoga class). Notice the sounds of the birds or crickets. Be mindful as you make love to your lover. Any practice of mindfulness can spill over into the other areas of your life. Immerse yourself in music, or feel the warm sun, the brisk refreshing cold, or a soothing breeze on your face. Can you be aware of life in all its subtlety? As you move your hand, can you notice the sensation of the air against your skin? When someone talks, can you appreciate not only the content but also the tone of the voice? Being aware of this type of subtlety can help you keenly focus on your present sensations.

⇨ Worrying about the Future

I am an old man and have known a great many troubles but most of them never happened.

MARK TWAIN

Anxiety over coming events, real or imagined, is a huge source of stress. Here, mindfulness can also be beneficial, but don't let it take the place of taking precautions for safety and security. Doing things like quitting smoking, installing and maintaining working fire alarms in your house, obtaining appropriate insurance, making wise financial plans, and regularly backing up your computer can alleviate a surprising amount of stress. If you still are preoccupied with the future, these worries can be dealt with in the same mindful fashion that we have previously discussed. Quickly and repeatedly, let each thought go, and focus on your diaphragmatic breath, muscle relaxation, or another present-moment sensation.

You may worry about your performance of a particular task. Yet when you examine a situation, it is clear that the worry only hampers your performance. Who would win a tennis match: the player obsessively worried about winning or the one focused on watching the ball and hitting the current shot? Skills being equal, the latter player would win. Whether you are making a business deal, raising children, or playing a sport, you will accomplish the task more efficiently and effectively if you focus on it, undistracted by your worries. Ironically, when you focus on the current process instead of the result, the result is usually better. It is important to have a good overall strategy, but obsessive worrying does not improve performance.

⇨ Process Reminder

When you find yourself obsessing or worrying about the results of a task, say to yourself, "Focus on the process; not the result." (Or you can shorten it to "process; not result.") This phrase will act as a reminder to bring your attention back to the work at hand—decreasing your stress and increasing both your performance and your enjoyment.

What if your mind is racing faster than a cheetah on steroids? Is there anything else you can do to deal with obsessive planning and worrying? Well, first off, there is no point in getting angry at your inherent tendency to plan. Consider the situation of a pending business deal in which you think of all the possible problems and dwell on how they should be handled. This process is analogous to the caveman's planning his defense from tigers or planning the best way to defeat a woolly mammoth. This tendency to plan helped the caveman stay alive. However, obsessing and dwelling on an issue adds to our stress. Fortunately, we have a tool that the earliest cavemen did not. We can write. Whether it be on paper or on the computer, we can write our plans down. There is less need to rehash the same stories over and over when the plan is already on paper.

✒ Put Your Plans on Paper

Instead of struggling against what you might feel is obsessive planning, write your plan down with the attitude that you are creating a great piece of artwork! Our minds have a natural tendency to strategize. Take pleasure in the art of creating a plan. Then you can enjoy your next activity.

"It's Too Hard" and "I'm Overwhelmed" Are Just Thoughts

Right now is a good time to remind you that you *can* successfully meditate and be mindful throughout the day. As people start exploring mindfulness, they sometimes think, "This is too hard," or "I can't do it." Here's the problem: When people start exploring mindfulness, they often expect to be able to stay focused on the present for 20 minutes without interruption. Then 1.8 seconds later comes the first distracting thought (perhaps something like "Look at what a great job I'm doing. Hey, I'm not focused on my breath. This is just too hard. I can't do anything right"). Newsflash: Don't expect to stay focused and mindful for an hour, 20 minutes, or even 20 seconds. Just one breath. That's all you need. When your mind drifts a thousand times, you gently bring it back a thousand times, just as you did earlier. So if you have the thought that mindfulness is too hard or if you think you need "peace of mind" or a "clear mind" before you can relax, remind yourself that those are just abstract concepts. All you need to do is let these thoughts go and enjoy the very next breath. Remember, even a small increase in mindfulness can mean a marked decrease in stress.

❖ The One-Breath Challenge

Let's do an experiment right now. On the count of 3, pay attention to one in breath and one out breath—that's right, just one breath. Ready, 1 . . . 2 . . . 3: go.

Were you able to do it? If not try again. OK. You've now demonstrated that you can be mindful without any problem. The next time you have a thought that it is difficult, you can let that thought go and fully focus on the next breath.

(For extra credit, here is one more short exercise: Start by picking out a muscle group that you would like to relax. On the count of 3, focus on your abdomen expanding with an in breath, and then with the out breath relax that muscle group. Ready, 1 . . . 2 . . . 3 . . . go.)

As you gain experience in meditation, you will soon appreciate its benefits. As things get stressful, you may think, "I need to modi tate," or "I need to clear my mind." If you are tense, meditation will likely help. However, the above thoughts suggest that your feelings are not OK as they are. They suggest that you need to change to be all right. I strongly recommend that people regularly meditate. However, before meditating out of a need, try just letting go of those thoughts and giving your full and complete attention to the full duration of an in breath and the full duration of an out breath (or another present-moment sensation). Being mindful takes only a moment and often gives you the perspective you need to deal with the stressful situation. You will find that if you then meditate with no immediate need or purpose, the meditation will be more fruitful.

Most of us have had the thought "I'm overwhelmed" at one time or another. Mindfulness teaches us to let that thought go and do what's next. For example, my first year of residency was one of my most stressful times. I might get called to see three people at once: Mr. A with shortness of breath, Mrs. B with chest pain, and Mr. C with leg pain. Rather than getting increasingly stressed, I let go of the thought "I'm overwhelmed" and focused my attention on taking care of one person at a time. I might ask Dr. Y to see Mr. A; then I would see Mrs. B, and then Mr. C. Alternatively, I might quickly check one patient to see that he was stable, then go to examine the next patient, and then return to the first. The point is to do what is next and focus on one thing at a time.

> Richard was feeling progressively more anxious and over-whelmed at work. He said that, at times, he felt like a "deer frozen in a car's headlights—too anxious to move." After we talked, Richard made a realistic plan of what he could accom-plish at work and prioritized the tasks. In addition, he planned to notice the thoughts that occurred when he felt stressed. He might notice the thought "I'm overwhelmed." As soon as he no-ticed that thought, he would let it go and focus on his breathing, taking slow, diaphragmatic breaths. If the thought "I'm over-whelmed" came up again, he would again, patiently, let it go. As time went on, Richard also noticed thoughts like "I don't like being here," "This is too hard," and "I hate this knot in my stom-ach." Each time he noticed one of these thoughts, he would let the thought go and focus on his breath. He would not resist the way his body felt. Instead of dwelling on everything he had to do, he would focus on doing the very next task. The more he did this, the more he found that he started enjoying his work and his stress decreased.

⊙ *Letting Go Meditation. Disk 1, Track 3.*
Length: 19 ½ Minutes

During this exercise, a variety of potentially stressful thoughts are introduced. However, by learning to let go of the thoughts, people invariably feel much more relaxed by the end of the meditation. This exercise clearly demonstrates that it is not the thoughts them-selves that cause stress, but what you do with the thoughts. There is another option besides believing and/or resisting all of your thoughts. Learning to mindfully let go of certain thoughts is an important step in learning to manage stress and to thrive in life.

Michele suffered from panic attacks. These attacks were so severe and disabling that she often used medication for them. Just the thought of having an anxiety attack could trigger one. As she was watching a ball game, a friend joked that a new soda had so much caffeine it might give him a panic attack. Michele then thought, "Oh no! What if I get a panic attack now? I don't have my medication with me! That would be horrible!"

Michele came into the office for a brief appointment to discuss the panic attacks. I had her start with focusing on diaphragmatic breaths. We did a meditation on breath. She started with letting go of her own thoughts. Then, I had her repeat the "charged thoughts" to herself (such as "Oh no! What if I get a panic attack now?"). Instead of fighting the thoughts, she was to notice them with interest. She watched how the thoughts would come and go. She was instructed to just notice any sensations with interest and not resist the sensations. When the exercise was over, she was surprised that despite thinking her most scary thoughts, she was actually very relaxed. She learned that those "scary thoughts" did not harm her at all. She did not have to push the thoughts away. The thoughts were, in fact, flimsy and harmless. It was how she had "charged" the thoughts that had created the problem. She had charged the thoughts by believing them, and trying to push them away/resist them. Developing the skill of mindfully noticing her thoughts helped her effectively deal with her panic attacks.

For as long as Justin could remember, he had had a problem with anxiety. One day, while he was under extreme stress, his heart

rate jumped to 180 beats per minute and he was diagnosed with
a heart rhythm problem called PSVT, or paroxysmal supraven-
tricular tachycardia. After that episode, his anxiety was far worse.
Although he never had another episode of PSVT, whenever his
heart rhythm was the least bit irregular he would start to panic.
As he panicked, the rhythm would become even more irregular
and uneven. Justin would start thinking, "I'm going to die; I hate
how I feel; I wish this would stop," and so on. It wasn't enough
for Justin to learn to relax. He needed to know how to deal with
his thoughts and physical sensations. We did a relaxation exercise
similar to the one on Disk 1, Track 3. He repeated the thoughts
that troubled him, but instead of resisting or believing the
thoughts, he practiced just mindfully noticing them. He then focused on a diaphragmatic breath. Now, in addition to the medicine his cardiologist recommended, he had a tool to deal with his
stress and did much better.

We are just beginning to explore the importance and the application of mindfulness. In the next chapter, you will learn hints to
make mindfulness a natural part of your day-to-day life. We'll discuss common barriers to mindfulness and simple ways to deal
with those barriers. Utilizing this information will decrease your
stress, improve your performance, and bring more joy to your day.

5

Put Mindfulness
into Practice

The secret of health for both mind and body is not to mourn for the past, not to worry about the future, nor to anticipate troubles, but to live the present moment wisely and earnestly.

BUDDHA

Reminders of Mindfulness

We have discussed how mindfulness is as simple as enjoying your next breath or feeling the ground massage your foot as you step. We have also discussed how increasing the frequency of these mindful episodes is a key to managing stress. What strategies, then, can we employ to increase the frequency of mindfulness?

In the last chapter, we recommended that as soon as you notice stress or a thought wishing the present to be different, you develop the reflex of letting the thought go and focusing on the present breath, footstep, and so on. (Also, consider relaxing a muscle group that you tend to tense under stress.)

An additional strategy is to assign certain events to be reminders to breathe mindfully. In his book *Peace Is Every Step*, Thich Nhat Hanh describes his experiences at a Buddhist monastery. Periodically throughout the day, a bell would ring. The sound of the bell was a signal to let any thoughts go and to enjoy the next breath. Now, when he hears a telephone ring, Hanh uses that sound as a reminder to enjoy the next breath instead of answering the phone immediately. Many of the occurrences that fill our day can be used as reminders to enjoy the present moment. Next time you are driving, decide that each red light will be a reminder to enjoy the next breath. For most people, a ringing telephone or red light is not a reminder of mindfulness. However, in order to increase mindful times throughout the day, we can consciously assign these events to be such reminders.

The sound of a beeper can be another reminder to breathe mindfully. Seeing the brake lights of the car in front of you could be a reminder. Another reminder might be a picture or a quotation posted on a wall.

On my office wall, I had a picture with the caption "Success is a journey, not a destination." Different quotations may have a special way of speaking to you. I ordered some coffee mugs with the saying "Take a little quiet time every day." As I drink my tea, I see another reminder.

Your daily routine can provide any number of reminders. A doctor's looking at the next patient's chart can be a signal to notice the next breath. As health care workers wash their hands between patients, their action can be a useful reminder to feel the soap and water, and to notice the fragrance of the hand lotion they might put on afterward. Having dishes to do can be a reminder to do a dishwashing meditation.

Sounds that are normally irritating can become reminders. If you are the parent of a baby, decide that each time the baby starts crying will be a reminder for you. It will be a signal to let go of thoughts wishing the present moment were different, to focus on your diaphragmatic breaths, and to relax a muscle group as you attend to your child's needs. You might doubt this approach can work during a stressful situation like caring for a crying baby. However, people use breathing exercises to deal with serious pain, including the pain of childbirth. They can work in almost any circumstance.

One of my patients made regular trips to the Xerox machine as part of her work. Each trip was her reminder. During work, another patient used Microsoft Outlook to schedule several times a day when a pop-up window on her computer would say, "Breathe." She would then take a one-minute break to focus on her breath. The morning alarm clock, an intermittent watch alarm, or the bell of a large clock can also be signals to let go of thoughts and to focus on the next breath. Another one of my class members took the stress management class with a coworker. Throughout the day they would just remind each other to breathe. One student bought a small timer that he wore on his belt. It either beeped or vibrated at regular intervals. Each time, he would take a mindful breath.

Many of us in the medical field enjoy seeing patients but dread paperwork and dictation. The small annoyance of a single dictation may not be a big deal, but if dictation is required 10 or 20 times a day, the frustration builds. Complete medical records are important for thorough patient care. If, instead of complaining, we would take that opportunity to enjoy a mindful breath, there would be 10 or 20 times that day that the stress could be decreased instead of increased. The instances add up.

Just reading through this section quickly may have minimal impact on your life. To make this technique more meaningful for you, take some time now to assign commonplace or everyday events to be reminders for you to take some mindful diaphragmatic breaths. Feel free to include the reminders mentioned above, and see if you can think of some additional ones. Refer to the list on a regular basis to ingrain the reminders into your mind.

If, several mornings in a row, you read a list that includes "car brake lights," you will soon think of mindful breathing as soon as you notice the brake lights of the car in front of you.

✎ Mindful Breathing Reminders

Write some reminders here, and add new reminders when you think of them. Think of a couple of reminders for different parts of your day—some to be used during work, some for home, and some for any other regular activities.

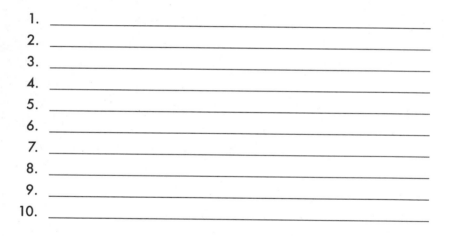

1. _____
2. _____
3. _____
4. _____
5. _____
6. _____
7. _____
8. _____
9. _____
10. _____

Let's say you've chosen at least three reminders of mindfulness and that one of them is red traffic lights. You review the reminders a few times, and later in the day, you actually are stopped by a red light as you are driving, but a wave of peacefulness does not spontaneously descend upon you from heaven. Don't immediately conclude, "This stuff doesn't work!" Being reminded is the beginning, not the end. When you see the red light, you must deliberately let any thoughts go and focus on taking a diaphragmatic breath. (Optionally, you can relax one of the muscle groups that you typically tense.)

Not My Job?

At one point, I was a little late in accomplishing a task. By the time I had gone back to do it, someone else had already done it. I apologized for causing him extra work. He kindly responded, "There is no extra work; just work." It was not a problem for him. Another person might have gotten more stressed by complaining to himself. My colleague just did the work mindfully, focusing on the task at hand.

Are there two artificial categories you make: work and extra work? Perhaps we focus on doing one part of a job with ease and even enjoy it. Then there is the extra work, and the thoughts come: "Somebody else should do this. It is not my responsibility. I hate the paperwork. I should not have to work this late." By obsessing with these thoughts, we create much distress. What if, instead, we told ourselves, "There is no extra work; just work?" We can let the thoughts go and focus on just enjoying the task at hand. That is not to say we should not try to change things. For instance, we might want to speak with a supervisor to change the required work, or we might want to delegate some of our work or figure out a way to decrease the paperwork. However, when we are right in the middle of required work, it helps to let go of the concept of "extra work" and just focus on the movement of our hand as we write, or the feeling of lifting the shovel as we dig.

✎ "Not My Job" List

Take some time now to note if there are tasks in your life that you make more difficult by thinking (in one form or another), "This is not my job"—that is, tasks that you tell yourself you would rather not do.

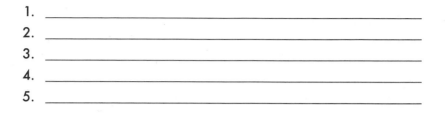

1. _____

2. _____

3. _____

4. _____

5. _____

Now, for each of those answers, take some time to reflect on two items: Would it be best to make plans to delegate this task, or is there another way that you should relieve yourself of this particular duty? If so, make plans to proceed along those lines.

It may be best that you continue with the task. It may take some time to relieve yourself of the duty. If either of these statements applies, each time you have the thought "This is not my job" or "I don't want to do this," let the thought go and do the task with your full attention and care. Just enjoy each small step. What are the small steps that make up the task? If you are ironing shirts, iron each sleeve with care. If you are washing dishes, wash one dish at a time. If you are dictating a report, dictate with care, one word at a time.

When Justification Becomes Rumination

The first temptation when you are anxious and stressed is to resist the stress and wish it away. We've reviewed how well that works—not very! We've also reviewed how wishing the circumstances of life were different can increase the distress. Let's say you really want to make things worse. What can you do next? Since most people haven't learned to accept feeling anxious or sad, there is a natural tendency to justify the emotions: "Hmm . . . I'm feeling anxious. Why is that?" And then you go on to list everything that could explain the anxiety. Now you can feel very justified in your anxiety. Do you see a problem here? Yes, listing all the things you could possibly be anxious about can only increase your anxiety.

"OK, OK," you're saying, "if I don't think about why I'm anxious, how can I correct it?" Good point. We do need to look at how we might improve our circumstances. However, it is very easy to go from solution-based thinking to counterproductive rumination. We need another alternative. And that, of course, brings us to mindfulness—learning to fully accept our emotions and physical sensations as they are.

> Samantha was participating in one of my stress reduction classes. She was having trouble with depression. I asked how she felt right now. She said she felt sad and wished she felt different. Since sadness was not an acceptable emotion for her, she always needed to find justifications for being sad. These included recent problems and problems from how she had been mistreated as a child. I asked if it was OK for her to let herself be sad. She said, "No. I hate being sad." I suggested that just for this moment, instead of resisting and justifying, she fully choose to feel whatever she felt. Then, 30 seconds later, I asked how she felt. She said, "Sad." Then, another 30 seconds later, I asked how she felt, and she no longer said, "Sad"; now she was relaxed. Usually her feelings of depression would last for hours. Samantha learned that trying to justify her feelings led to rumination and more depression. Instead, she could learn to be mindful.

It's time to further define mindfulness.

Defining Mindfulness

The Guest-House
This being human is a guest-house.

Every morning a new arrival.
A joy, a depression, a meanness,
some momentary awareness comes
as an unexpected visitor.
Welcome and entertain them all!
Even if they're a crowd of sorrows,
who violently sweep your house
empty of its furniture,
still, treat each guest honorably.
He may be clearing you out
for some new delight.
The dark thought, the shame, the malice,
meet them at the door laughing,
and invite them in.
Be grateful for whoever comes,
because each has been sent
as a guide from beyond.
   —RUMI

Now that you may have some sense of mindfulness, let's formally define it. Mindfulness is moment-to-moment nonjudgmental awareness. Its qualities include being flexible and fluid. The opposite of the flexibility of mindfulness is clinging to an idea and/or feeling of how things should be different. At times, this clinging is obvious; at other times, subtle. Even without thoughts of wanting the present to be different, we can sometimes sense the clinging. I was walking around with my sons, who were dawdling as only four-year-olds can, and I noticed a sense of irritation beginning to arise in me. Subconsciously, I was clinging to my desire that the boys should move more quickly. As soon as I noticed it, I stopped clinging. Although I was a little hungry, I was not on a deadline. I noted the feeling of hunger without pushing it away. If I chose to, I could still encourage my boys to hurry, but without the irritation caused from the clinging. Since we were not in a rush, I just assumed their slower pace and enjoyed our walk.

An important aspect of mindfulness is a curious or interested quality; we pay attention to each little detail of a sensation, emotion, or thought. Instead of comparing one bite of food to the next, we appreciate each bite as a unique moment. I give lots of lectures and usually am pretty comfortable speaking in front of groups. One day, I attended a professional conference. As it was my turn to speak and the microphone approached, my heart started racing. Instead of trying to hide this feeling or push it away, I just became very interested. My heart did not usually race as I spoke to groups. I let myself be curious and fully enjoyed and experienced the sensation. Before long my heart stopped pounding and I felt very comfortable and relaxed.

Author and Zen master Shunryu Suzuki describes mindfulness as having a "beginner's mind." When we experience an event with this beginner's mind, we do not get bored. Even if we have done something 100 times before, we can experience it with the interest and curiosity we have for a new experience. Just as a young child walks barefoot on the grass for the first time with awe and wonder, we can also enjoy each step.

Mindfulness has an affectionate or embracing quality. We welcome any new sensation, thought, or emotion. When we welcome all "visitors," we still cry in sadness, but without the tension of resisting an "unwelcome" emotion. And the very next moment will be something new. Will it be another variation of sadness or happiness, or something else? Whatever the case, it will be a unique moment, and our words will not really be able to fully describe it. Let's be curious to meet this new, unique moment and welcome each new "visitor."

Jim was very uneasy at the beginning of our first visit. He eventually revealed that the main reason for the visit was a problem with sex. For the most part, his life was going well. He had recently married and had previously enjoyed an active sex life with his wife. A month before our meeting, however, he had been particularly stressed and unable to attain an erection. Ever since that time, either he hadn't been able to attain an erection during sex, or if he had, he'd lost it quickly.

Since Jim did have normal erections when he woke up at night, I suspected that the primary problem was psychological stress. Like most men, Jim had had an experience in which he had been unable to have an erection. Instead of shrugging it off as something that most men experience on occasion, Jim had become very worried about it. The next time he'd had sex, all he could think about was whether his erection would occur, so, of course, it did not. If he did get an erection, he would fixate on how it was doing. Normally, the intensity of an erection waxes and wanes during sex. But with Jim's anxiety about it, he would panic as soon as his erection was less intense, and then he'd lose the erection altogether.

After our visit, Jim worked with the meditations on Disk 1. He learned to gently let distracting thoughts go and put his attention on his wife instead of his erection. He let go of any goal and paid full attention to and enjoyed the present-moment sensations. Each time his mind wandered, he patiently brought his attention back to the present. He focused on each kiss as if it was their first; he noted the variety of subtle sensations that came from just one touch. He did not cling to any goal and he embraced each sensation just as it was. At our follow-up visit, three weeks later, Jim's problem was much better, despite his unfilled prescription for Viagra.

Make Emotions Simple

In order to mindfully experience a particular moment, it helps to accurately attend to the moment. Consider, for instance, the description "I feel horribly empty." It might be very difficult to be mindful if we think that we feel "horribly empty." How can we not resist or judge such a feeling? But what if we try to accurately and nonjudgmentally describe it instead? If we look at "I feel horribly empty," we may see the emotion is sadness; physically, there might be a tight feeling in the abdomen, and then we may have a series of thoughts such as "I feel horribly empty," "I can't take this any longer," and/or "I hope I feel better soon." When we mindfully register the sadness, it is fully experienced—and in the next moment, we are open to the next emotion. Perhaps it will be another shade of sadness; perhaps anger; perhaps joy. We are not stuck with being sad about being sad. We can then mindfully accept the physical sensation. (Even painful physical sensations are not as bothersome when they are mindfully attended to. This is why mindfulness training has been very useful for patients in chronic pain.)

As we pay keen attention to our emotions, we can observe that what we sometimes call an emotion is rather a thought, or a combination of emotion and thought. For instance, when we are meditating, we might say, "I feel like getting up now." It is probably more accurate to say, "I felt a tightness in my abdomen and had the thought that I wanted to get up." Then we can be mindful of the abdominal tightness and notice the thought as a thought. Similarly, when we are frustrated, we might say, "I feel like escaping." This reaction might be described as "I feel anger or frustration and I had the thought 'I feel like escaping.'" Another example is "I feel overwhelmed." Likely, this could more accurately be described as "I feel anxious and have the thought that I am overwhelmed." Still another example is "I feel like having a cigarette." In that case, we could describe the thought of "I feel like having a cigarette" and investigate the true associated physical sensations and emotions.

When you are stuck, a useful exercise is to chart out (on paper or just in your mind) the basic components of your experience. Break the experience into emotion, physical sensations, and thoughts. You might try using just the five emotions of happiness, sadness, anger, peacefulness, and high energy ("high energy" encompassing both anxiety and excitement, as in our earlier discussion of eustress*). Even what is considered a common emotion such as loneliness can be examined more closely. Loneliness can be thought of as sadness with an implied series of thoughts about wanting to be with another person. If you wanted to use the five categories of emotion listed above, you might list frustration as anger with an implication that you wish something were different.

When you start talking or thinking about more complicated emotions, see if you can more accurately describe the thoughts, emotions, and physical sensations that are involved. When you say, "I'm empty," what does your body feel like? Perhaps there is heaviness around your eyes. Is the emotion sadness? What thoughts are there? Paying this type of close attention can help you become more mindful and not just lost in your thoughts.

---

*As described in Chapter 4, when we closely observe anxiety, we may note that the physical sensations themselves are similar to excitement. With anxiety, we usually have thoughts wishing that our physical sensations and/or our external situation were different. With excitement, the adrenaline still flows and the heart still races, but we are enjoying the adrenaline flow, not resisting it.

✎ Mindfulness Chart

When you feel stuck sometime, see if you can fill in the chart with some other examples. Feel free to make your own chart if you run out of room.

Situation	Physical Sensations	Emotion	Thoughts
Have not heard from my friend	Tightness in neck	Sadness	I feel lonely. I wish my friend were here.
Work is very busy	Abdomen is tense	High energy	I feel overwhelmed. Work is too busy. I wish I didn't work here.

Accurately describing our emotions, physical sensations, and thoughts enhances our ability to be mindful.

Derek was a scientist. He had a terribly frustrating time when he tried to meditate. I asked Derek not to try to relax. I explained that trying too hard to relax could just make the relaxation more difficult. I advised him just to pay attention to his breathing and told him that when he noticed his attention drifting, he could be thankful for the moment of noticing and bring his attention back. If his mind drifted a million times the job was to patiently bring his attention back a million and one times. I used a science analogy. Instead of trying to relax, the meditation was just a research experiment. He could notice, with curiosity, what thoughts, sensations, and emotions came to his awareness. Even if he had a thought of being bored, he could notice that thought with curiosity. I advised him not to judge the thoughts as good or bad, but to notice them with the curiosity of a scientist. After all, during a normal day he might be too distracted to pay this close attention to his thoughts, sensations, and emotions. The meditation was his time set aside for this careful research.

Derek used a microscope during his normal science job. I explained how he could use the microscope of "bare attention" to closely observe what was happening in his awareness. When he noted his thoughts as thoughts, his emotions as emotions, and his physical sensations, he could learn to mindfully accept whatever came into his present awareness. After this discussion, Derek meditated faithfully for 40 minutes each morning, enjoying it as a special time to research an extremely important subject: his own awareness, how he caused his own suffering, and how to relieve his suffering.

Noting

Noting your thoughts, emotions, and physical sensations as they arise is a tool you can use to foster mindfulness. For instance, you can say words to yourself like *sadness, thought,* or *neck tightness* as one of those events happens. At times, this process may help you focus your attention more easily and see how your thoughts, emotions, and physical sensations come and go. Author and Buddhist teacher Jack Kornfield states that this noting should be subtle and soft, and at most 5 percent of the experience. Most of the time is spent fully experiencing each phenomenon.

Most important, this noting is not complaining. The noting is done in a welcoming fashion. Kornfield has used the phrase "bowing to" the sensation, thought, and/or emotion. If you like, you can even try getting more specific about the particular type of thought. For instance, if you are obsessing, you could say, "Obsessing" or "Obsessing mind." At times, you may be stressed because of the effort of comparing yourself to another, and you could note, "Comparing" or "Competitive mind." If you are complaining to yourself about extra work, you could note, "Complaining." Again, the noting is not a criticism. Sometimes, you may even feel as if you're telling yourself an inside joke, or perhaps saying hello to an old friend.

Noting might have the feel of playing a fun game of tag with a child. There is one difference, however. After my five-year-old sons tag me, I let them do their "na na na na na" dance (the one where they put their thumbs in their ears, wiggle their fingers, and stick out their tongues while wiggling their hips). Then I run around a bit, letting them get away, and then finally I tag them. With mindfulness, don't let the thought or sensation dance and run around for too long. Note it as soon as you realize it is there. Still, note it in the same lighthearted fashion as a game of tag with a child. Noting is an optional

At one point, "thought stopping" was a popular psychological technique. To deal with obsessive thoughts, it was recommended that people try to stop the thoughts. People would even wear a rubber band on their wrists and snap it when they had the thought. Here is the problem: Even the term *thought stopping* creates an antagonistic mind-set. It implies that one needs to get rid of thoughts. For many, this works as well as carrying water in a spaghetti strainer. In other words, resisting our thoughts can lead to frustration and more stress. The process of noting is not thought stopping. With noting we assume a friendly, welcoming attitude to our thoughts, sensations, and emotions. When we don't try to stop or push away thoughts, and instead mindfully note them, they do a fine job of drifting by on their own.

tool, and you can see if it helps you to become more mindful, both during your formal meditation sessions and with experiences throughout the day.

Recent scientific research supports the practice of noting. One recent study used functional MRI brain scans to demonstrate a mechanism by which putting feelings into words helps reduce distress.

A Relaxation "Quickie"

In Western culture, we tend to think of the mind and the body as separate. However, distress manifests with both mental agitation and muscular tension. As we calm our minds, our muscles will usually relax, and as we calm our muscles, our minds will often become more focused. Therefore, combining a technique for focusing the mind with a technique for relaxing your muscles can be very effective in dealing with your distress. If you do not have time for a long sitting or walking meditation, try this interesting and effective exercise to quickly reduce your level of stress.

❖ Muscle-Relaxation Meditation

This exercise is useful since it can be done quickly and in any posture: sitting, standing, or lying down. With each inhalation, notice your abdomen gently go out. With each exhalation, relax a different muscle group. For instance, with the first exhalation, you might relax your jaw; with the second, your neck; with the third, the little muscles between your eyes; with the fourth, your shoulders; and with the fifth exhalation, your back. You may try another muscle group, such as your arms or legs. It will not be long until you are feeling more relaxed.

The Three-Minute Breathing Space

During one of my stress management classes, a participant asked if there were any questions he could ask himself to become more mindful. After some thought, I recommended three: (1) What physical sensations do I feel now? (2) What emotion am I feeling now? and (3) What thoughts am I having now? In essence, one must start where one is. Zindel Segal, Mark Williams, and John Teasdale developed a class called mindfulness-based cognitive therapy, or MBCT. This class was developed to decrease the frequency with which people relapse into clinical depression. After participating in MBCT, students who had had three or more episodes of depression had a 44 percent decreased chance of relapse. One technique that participants were taught was the three-minute breathing space.

❖ *The Three-Minute Breathing Space*
1. **During the** first minute, just assess what is going on currently: What are your specific physical sensations, emotions, and thoughts? Do not try to change the sensations, emotions, and thoughts; just mindfully note them.
2. **During the** second minute, turn your full attention to your breath. Again, focus on the full duration of the in breath and the full duration of the out breath. Note where the breath seems easy to follow, perhaps at the nostrils or in the abdomen as it expands.
3. **For the** third minute, expand your awareness to include your body. Be aware of your whole body in the process of breathing.

In addition to longer periods of meditation, MBCT participants are advised to use the three-minute breathing space three times a day and also as needed. Keep in mind that you can use the ideas behind this technique for a shorter or longer "breathing space." Whether it's ten seconds or thirty minutes, it can be beneficial.

Choosing Each Moment to Train Your Brain

In Spring, hundreds of flowers,
In Autumn, a harvest moon,
In Summer, a refreshing breeze,
In Winter, snow will accompany you.
If useless things do not hang in your mind,
Any season is a good season for you.

MUMON EKAI

Notice that the poem does not say, "If useless things do not come to your mind." It says *hang* in your mind: How we deal with the thoughts that we have can bring us back to enjoying the present moment. Put another way:

That the birds fly overhead, this you cannot stop. That they build a nest in your hair, this you can prevent.

ANCIENT CHINESE PROVERB

Some of you may remember Roseanne Roseannadanna from the television show *Saturday Night Live.* She had the catch phrase "It's always something." I have found that, at any given moment, if I choose to, I can be creative enough to find something to be stressed about. If we choose not to be mindful, there is indeed "always something." If I try hard enough, I can always worry about some future situation, worry that I have acted inappropriately in the past, or wish that the present moment were different. At any given moment, I have the choice of whether I will dwell on these thoughts or enjoy the present.

Our thoughts of discontent may seem to be unique, but they are usually nothing really special. They are likely to be very similar to thoughts we have had in our past and will have in our future. Within each moment is a test of how you want to spend that moment and, as the moments add up, how you want to spend your life.

Think of a cart on a soft dirt road. Each time it travels the same path, the rut in the dirt gets deeper. Each time you focus on how the present moment should be different, you not only suffer in that moment but also strengthen this habit of thinking. However, when you take a new path—the path of enjoying this very moment—you strengthen that path.

As we learn more about the brain, this analogy becomes more meaningful. Scientists now feel that the brain has a significant amount of neuroplasticity. That is, the structure of the brain is always changing. As in a freeway network, new routes are created and improved with use, while old, low-traffic routes are abandoned. Each time we choose to be mindful, we create stronger neural pathways that become easier to follow.

⇨ Choosing Mindfulness

When you find yourself obsessing over a problem, ask yourself if this one issue is worth a life of distress. Wouldn't you rather have one of enjoyment? Set the precedent for how to handle the thoughts and issues in your life now. The only time you can choose to be mindful is right now. Do not waste this moment; choose mindfulness!

Cultivating Mindfulness

I went to the woods because I wished to live deliberately, to front only the essential facts of life, and see if I could not learn what it had to teach, and not, when I came to die, discover that I had not lived.

HENRY DAVID THOREAU

Henry David Thoreau went to the woods, in essence, to cultivate mindfulness. What are the things we can do at home to practice living deliberately, fully, and mindfully? In addition to reading about mindfulness, it is important to develop an experiential understanding of mindfulness. Mindfulness is not something to be learned once and then forgotten. It is to be continually remembered and cultivated. What follows are exercises that should increase your experiential understanding of mindfulness. Additionally, as you repeat the exercises, you will further cultivate your ability to be mindful.

Remember that our brains can be changed with the right type of training. Scientists used to think that each of us had a happiness set point that was fairly unchangeable. We win the lottery and get happier for a little while, and then our emotional state gradually returns to the set point. Something bad happens and our happiness decreases, only to come back to the baseline with time. Now we know that just as we can change our biceps by practicing curls with a barbell, we can change our brains with the exercises below. Think of them as mental curls. By using these exercises (and exercises described in Chapter 11), we can actually raise our happiness set point, so we can thrive during the ups and downs of life.

As we learn about and cultivate mindfulness, we also make wiser choices. We find more "space" between a stimulus and a reaction. Instead of reacting automatically to stress, we can mindfully notice our thoughts, feelings, and emotions and then make a wiser choice on how to act.

To summarize, through cultivating mindfulness, we can be happier, less stressed, and make better choices. Sound good? I thought so. Plan to do at least one of the exercises below per day as you continue your journey through this book.

The exercises on the CDs contain a lot of instruction and guidance. This will help you effectively learn the techniques. Once you get the hang of the guided exercises, the non-guided exercises can be done on your own. For the latter, no CD player is needed, so you can do them whether you're hiking in the wilderness or just having a few free minutes at work.

⊙ *Sound, Breath, Body, Thoughts & Emotions. Disk 1, Track 4. Length: 21¹/₂ Minutes*

Traditional exercises to cultivate mindfulness include attending to your breath, body sensations, sounds, thoughts, and emotions. Listen to the track, letting it lead you through mindfulness of each of these areas. This meditation starts with a very brief "relaxation quickie" or "muscle relaxation meditation" as described earlier in this chapter.

It is also beneficial to spend a whole meditation session on just one object of attention. This process is described in more depth below.

In all of these exercises, when your attention drifts, return it nonjudgmentally. The following exercises are flexible in length. They can be practiced from 5 to 40 minutes. (As you begin, a length of 5 to 10 minutes is probably enough.)

❖ *Breath Meditation*

In Chapter 3, we talked in some depth about *awareness of breath.* The breath is always with us (at least as long as we are alive).

Therefore, breathing meditation is a convenient tool to strengthen our focus and attention. Optionally, try noting "rising" and "falling" with each breath. Suggested time: 5 to 40 minutes.

❖ Body Sensations Meditation

Focus on your breath as you open your awareness to physical sensations. As you pay close attention to your body, you will note the subtleties. There may be pain, throbbing, itching, or warmth. The sensations may get more or less intense when they are closely observed. What does become clear is that the sensations continually change. Experiment to see what it is like to sit with your body sensations nonjudgmentally. (Of course, some sensations need to be acted upon, but many do not.) Suggested time: 5 to 20 minutes.

❖ Sound Meditation

Pay attention to sound while nonjudgmentally letting go of your thoughts. You may be surprised by your experience. Let go of the tendency to label the sounds as good or bad. As you listen for all the subtlety, can you hear the music in the mundane? Can you appreciate not only the birds chirping, but also the traffic noise or the water in the sink? Instead of distractions, let those sounds be your focus. Suggested time: 5 to 20 minutes.

❖ Thought Meditation

Let your thoughts be the subject of your awareness rather than a distraction. Instead of being lost in the content of your thoughts, try just observing them as if they were going across a video screen. You might notice as you try to focus on your thoughts that there are no thoughts to focus on. If that's the case, just focus on the space between the thoughts. Suggested time: 5 to 10 minutes.

❖ Choiceless Awareness

Cultivate mindfulness of whatever comes into your awareness, be it your breath, a physical sensation, a sound, a smell, a taste, a thought, or an emotion. This process has been termed *choiceless awareness*. In a way, this type of meditation most closely mimics day-to-day life. You nonjudgmentally observe whatever comes into your awareness. You can notice how each sensation, thought, or emotion arises and passes. One way to explore choiceless awareness is to first focus on your breath, and then to expand your awareness to include your body as well. Then expand it to include sounds and then all your senses. Try resting in the "space" of all that comes into your awareness.

Other names for this type of meditation include insight, mindfulness, or vipassana meditation. An advantage of this style of meditation is that it most closely replicates being mindful in day-to-day life. However, your ability to do insight meditation is strengthened by developing your concentration with the four previous meditations.

Suggested time: 5 to 40 minutes.

For the exercise below, you can have the CD guide you through the exercise and later do it on your own at your own pace.

◉ Walking Meditation. Disk 1, Track 5. Length: 4 Minutes

Listen to this exercise in a place where you have at least a space of 10 feet in which you can walk. It will introduce you to walking meditation. When we walk from, say, one office to another, do we use the time to stress about work, or could the time be used to become more relaxed and joyful? There are two ways to do a walking meditation. I suggest you practice both. One way is to bring your focus back to the sensation only in the lower part of your body—your legs and your feet. Everything else is in the background. During each footstep, you focus on the feeling of lifting and placing your foot. You can focus on feeling your foot on the ground. If it is helpful, some of the time you can try saying, "Lifting," as you lift your foot, and "Placing," as you place your foot down. The focus of a walking meditation is not on getting somewhere, but on being present with each step. It has been described as "arriving in each step." Some of my students have found it useful to say to themselves with each step, "Arrived." As you let yourself enjoy each step, you may even feel the purposeful placement of each foot as a slow dance. One difference is you do not have to learn any fancy dance step.

After you have practiced the first style of walking meditation, you may also want to practice walking meditation with the sense of "choiceless awareness." Then, in addition to the sensation of your legs, you can open your awareness to sounds, breath, vision, touch (the feel of the wind or sun on your skin), and so on.

⊙ *Eating Meditation. Disk 2, Track 1. Length: 7 Minutes*

Listen to this exercise as you are about to sit down to a meal. Most of us unconsciously eat most of our meals—in essence, cultivating indigestion instead of mindfulness. With so much food eaten unconsciously, no wonder there is an epidemic of obesity in the United States. What difference would it make if most of those meals were eaten mindfully? The eating meditation will be discussed further in Chapter 9.

⊙ *Stretching Meditation. Disk 2, Track 2. Length: 8 Minutes*

For your convenience, this series of mindful stretches is designed to be done in a chair, so you can do this exercise when you have just eight minutes free at work or home. With stretching meditation or yoga, can you feel your breath as you move? Can you let go of thoughts and have your attention in your body? If you are exerting one area of your body, can you allow the other areas to soften and relax? Once you feel comfortable with this exercise, you may chose to participate in a longer stretching or yoga program.

When describing formal meditation practice, Jon Kabat-Zinn uses the metaphor of weaving a parachute. You do not want to start weaving your parachute as you jump out of the plane. It helps to have worked on the parachute prior to the flight. In the same way, the formal meditation practice allows you to practice dealing with your thoughts and emotions prior to a stressful event. In addition to the CDs, most people benefit from a more formal class or training in mindfulness. One widely taught health class in the United States is called mindfulness-based stress reduction, or MBSR. There are also other types of classes in mindfulness meditation. One of the advantages of MBSR is that the curriculum has been somewhat standardized. Additionally, the curriculum has been subjected to scientific research, which shows improvement in anxiety and chronic pain. For more information on mindfulness classes, see "Recommended Web Sites" at the end of this book, or find this and other useful information on my Web site www.stressremedy.com.

Summary

   I. Mindfulness is moment-to-moment nonjudgmental awareness. To practice mindfulness:

A. Let go of thoughts about how the present moment should be different. These include thoughts about how your body should feel different and/or how your particular circumstances should be different.

B. Focus on the present moment. It is particularly effective to focus on your breath and, even better, to breathe using your diaphragm. It is also effective to focus on any present input into your senses, such as taste, touch, smell, vision, and hearing.

II. Notice if certain muscle groups tend to get tense during stressful times. If so, as soon as stress becomes apparent, do Steps A and B described above, and then focus your attention on those muscle groups. Allow the muscles to relax just as you did in the meditation. Do not resist the sensations. Relaxing a particular muscle group is easiest if you do it as soon as you notice the stress.

III. Ideally, the above steps should be done quickly. As soon as a thought of resistance appears, let it go. Do not let the cycle of stress go on for long.

IV. The above steps should be done repetitively and regularly. Mindfulness is a lifetime practice and a lifetime challenge. Each resistant thought you have gives you more opportunity to practice letting these thoughts go. When first learning about mindfulness, many are surprised by how much of the time they are not mindful. But keep in mind: Even a small increase in the amount of time that you are mindful can dramatically improve the way you handle stress.

V. Continue to set goals for the future. In certain cases, changing your external environment is an extremely important way to deal with stress. However, realize that the present can be only the way it is. It is essential to learn to enjoy the process of change.

VI. Learn to use your energy, instead of resisting it.

VII. Take appropriate precautions for your future, and use mindfulness to deal with worrying.

VIII. Mindfulness skills can be used to deal with habitual behaviors.

IX. Focus on doing one thing at a time.

X. Assign certain events to be reminders to breathe mindfully.

XI. Ask the questions "What are the physical sensations? What is the emotion? What are the thoughts?" It is easier to be mindful when we do not confuse our thoughts with emotions.

XII. Optionally, you can use subtle noting to help focus your awareness.

XIII. Meditate regularly and, if possible, daily. Practicing regular meditation increases your tendency to be mindful throughout the day. Remember the exercises above. Do at least one a day as you explore the rest of the book.

XIV. Consider further reading and courses to hone and cultivate your mindfulness skills.

🖉 Chapter Review

What are your thoughts about mindfulness?

What did you learn from doing the CD exercises?

6

Change Your Thoughts

IN 1955, THE psychologist Albert Ellis began popularizing the field of cognitive therapy. He came up with the ABCs of how our thoughts affect our emotions. He referred to an event that happens as the "antecedent," or A. The event is often followed by an emotional "consequence," or C. For instance, A might be your boss yelling at you. C, the consequence, would be that you become upset. Or A might be that your favorite team wins the Superbowl, and C would be that you feel overjoyed. A causes C, right?

Not so fast. The reason you got so upset or overjoyed was not the antecedent (A), but the set of "beliefs," which we'll call B, that you used to interpret the event, and that created your emotional response. To summarize, A (the antecedent) triggers B (the beliefs), which in turn triggers C (the consequence). The antecedent doesn't cause your emotion; your interpretation of it does—and, as Ellis showed, our interpretations are often irrational. Perhaps when your boss yelled, you had a series of thoughts: "I can't do anything right. . . . I'll probably get fired. . . . I'll never get another job. . . . He probably thinks I'm a total failure." A yelling boss may be annoying, but he can't make you feel miserable unless your irrational beliefs do their part.

Ellis recommended adding a D to the ABCs, suggesting that we can and should "dispute" the irrational beliefs. In the above example, such D thoughts might include "I made one mistake; that does not mean I do everything wrong"; "I've done most of my work correctly, and I doubt that I'd get fired for doing one thing wrong"; "If I did get fired, it might be a little difficult, but I'd find another job"; "He just yelled at me today. Maybe he is having a bad day. I know that when I yell at somebody, it has more to do with my inner frustration than anything else." Disputing the irrational beliefs usually decreases stress, anger, frustration, and sadness.

Of course, in order to dispute the irrational beliefs, we have to recognize them as such—and that means labeling them. As the field of cognitive therapy developed, the irrational beliefs we all have came to be known as *cognitive distortions*. Thoughts clouded with cognitive distortions make viewing the world as if through a cloudy, distorted lens. The cognitive distortions cause situations to seem worse than they really are. But once you become aware of the distorted lenses you are wearing, you can take them off and see each situation clearly. By categorizing irrational beliefs, we more easily recognize them. In his book *Feeling Good*, the psychiatrist David Burns discusses nine categories of cognitive distortion:

- **All-or-none thinking.** If you do not perform perfectly, you think of yourself as a total failure.
- **Overgeneralization.** If one thing goes wrong, you start thinking, "Nothing goes right."

○ **Magnification or catastrophizing.** One simple mishap is interpreted as the end of the world.

○ **Minimization.** You ignore a variety of things that have gone right for you.

○ **Labeling.** One or two relationships do not work out, so you consider yourself unlovable. Something goes wrong at one job and you decide you are worthless. If other people's behavior disturbs you, you label them jerks, rather than trying to understand their point of view.

○ **Personalization.** You blame yourself for an event that was not your fault. For instance, it is not uncommon for a child to blame herself for her parents' divorce.

○ **Emotional reasoning.** You assume that, because you feel bad, you are bad. An example would be thinking, "I feel sad and worthless. Therefore, I must be worthless."

○ **Jumping to conclusions:**
   ~ **Mind reading.** You assume that you know what another person is thinking. The person who did not return your call must be mad at you. The person who is giggling must be laughing at you.
   ~ **Fortune-telling.** You upset yourself by predicting the worst possible outcome for the future.

○ **"Should" statements.** You dwell in the past, thinking about how you should have acted differently.

It's easy to see the distortions in these thinking patterns. For instance, we all have 20/20 vision in hindsight, which isn't available to us as we make our choices. Accept your past decisions and move on. Learning from our mistakes is a key part of personal development, but obsessing on them helps no one. Let go of any "should" conversations as soon as you notice them. The only "should" question that might be useful to ask is "How should I act now or in the future?"

When first learning to recognize cognitive distortions, it helps to categorize them and chart them on paper. Just writing down an irrational belief often allows you to see how truly irrational it is. Let's apply this technique to the earlier example:

Situation	Emotions	Automatic Thoughts	Type of Cognitive Distortion	Dispute (Rational Response)
Your boss yells at you.	Sadness, anger	"I can't do anything right."	All-or-none thinking	"I did one thing wrong, but I've done a lot right."
	Frustration	"He probably thinks that I'm a total failure."	Mind-reading	"He had a short fuse today. I can't assume that he thinks poorly of me."

Now let's look at an example from one of my patients:

When I first saw Mary, she had recurring episodes of stress and depression that would last for months. The episodes seemed more understandable once we had reviewed some of the thoughts that typically accompanied these periods. As soon as she would start feeling depressed, Mary would think, "Oh, no! Here I go again—another two months of stress and depression." At these times, Mary would often focus on a recent past relationship in which she had been abused. She would think, "I never should have stayed in that relationship. I can't maintain a good relationship. I feel really down. I'm worthless." We talked about the impact of cognitive distortions, and Mary made the following chart. She began to see the patterns that had worsened her stress and depression. This recognition made it easier for her to shift her thinking.

Emotions	Thoughts	Type of Cognitive Distortion	Dispute
Stress Anxiety Depression	"Another two months of stress."	Fortune telling	That happened in the past, but not necessarily now. Let's reimagine the situation and make it a challenge to have this episode be much shorter.
	"I never should have stayed in that relationship."	Should statement	Instead of berating myself, I will focus on the lessons that I learned in the relationship. For instance, I will not tolerate abuse in future relationships.
	"I can't maintain a good relationship."	All-or-none thinking	I made mistakes in past relationships, but I learned from them.
	"I feel really down. I'm worthless."	Emotional reasoning	Just because I feel bad does not mean that I am bad or worthless.

As you gain experience in quickly recognizing cognitive distortions, charting them will usually not be necessary. All are variations on the theme of magnifying the negative aspects of a situation and minimizing the positive ones.

When you find yourself making general statements about a problem or failure, it is helpful to dispute the generalization. Saying strongly negative phrases to yourself or to others can dramatically increase your stress. On the other hand, putting situations into a more rational perspective can help alleviate the stress. (This topic is described further in Chapter 8.)

Simply replacing strongly negative phrases with less forceful or dramatic phrases can help with stress as well. Typical catastrophizing may include thoughts such as "This is horrible"; "What a catastrophe"; "I'm ruined"; "This is a nightmare"; and "I can't believe it happened." Have you ever said any of those things to yourself? Think about how your stress would decrease if you replaced those phrases with the milder and more accurate phrase "That was unfortunate." *Unfortunate* is a very useful addition to your mental vocabulary. Another strategy is to ask if a problem will really matter in 10 years.

> Denise worked setting up displays at a store. One day, she had spent all day setting up a display exactly as she had been instructed. At the end of the day, her boss changed her mind about what she wanted. Denise was very upset. She found herself thinking, "This is horrible! I can't believe this happened." When she realized that she was catastrophizing, she corrected herself in a way that was much closer to the truth: "It's inconvenient that I will have to set up a new display." Once she realized that the situation was not the "end of the world," she felt much better and stopped working herself into a frenzy.

In time, you will automatically recognize cognitive distortions and quickly act to dispel them. Another way to decrease your stress is through a technique called *reframing*.

Reframing

Reframing involves placing a particular situation in a new frame or context. By doing so, you don't change the situation itself, but you change your interpretation of it, and thus your stress response to it. Initially, you might view a difficult task as an objectionable chore. By reframing, you can view the task as an enjoyable challenge. Now, you may think that there is only one appropriate response to any particular situation, but that wasn't the conclusion of two men who found numerous occasions to reframe their highly public lives:

We are continually faced by great opportunities brilliantly disguised as insoluble problems.

LEE IACOCCA

The pessimist sees difficulty in every opportunity. The optimist sees opportunity in every difficulty.

WINSTON CHURCHILL

Thomas Edison worked long, hard hours and failed in many of his attempts to invent the incandescent lightbulb. These failed attempts would have discouraged many people. However, Edison said, "I am not discouraged, because every wrong attempt discarded is another step forward."

How many times have we berated ourselves for not doing something correctly, or sometimes even for not doing something perfectly? Instead of interpreting an effort as a failure, it's much more productive to reframe an unsuccessful effort as an opportunity to learn.

Unsatisfying interactions with others can also be reframed as opportunities to learn. Few things are more stressful than having someone be rude to you. Whether it's at the bank or Aunt Martha's house, it sends your blood pressure right through the roof. But a little reflection can change all that. In my stress management classes, I always ask, "Who here has ever been rude?" Typically, all the participants raise their hands. Next I ask, "When you have been rude, is it usually when you are happy and feeling your best?" The unanimous answer is no. This unofficial study yields very convincing results. If fifty out of fifty people in class after class are suffering in some way when they are rude, then perhaps we can extrapolate further: When people act rude, they are probably suffering, too. Bear this in mind when an acquaintance is rude. Instead of immediately reacting with anger, realize that he or she may not be doing well. Did the bank teller's wife just file for divorce? Did your boss just find out about her sister's breast cancer?

Much of our communication is with people we don't know well. We know very little about what is going on in their lives and their minds—the "tip of the iceberg." Even with close friends and family, we can't know all of the issues that may be troubling them. If people are rude, almost undoubtedly they are unhappy. At times, it may be helpful to ask if something is bothering them. Other times, it might only inflame the situation. In either case, it decreases your own stress and hostility to appreciate that the surface rudeness probably stems from a deeper suffering that has little to do with you.

What about the people who seem to be rude most of the time? Well, perhaps they are unhappy most of the time. Perhaps they are clinically depressed or are in chronic pain. Also, remember that rudeness may simply spring from a difference in communication styles. For instance, a fast-talking person may seem rude to someone not accustomed to such brusqueness.

I once called a business associate and a woman answered the telephone in a shockingly rude manner. She asked, "Why the (blank) are you calling again?" I was stunned but asked to speak with my associate. She refused to take a message or to give me another way to reach him. I was tempted to give her some of her own rude medicine. Instead, I told myself that she must be having a really, really bad day, that her rudeness had nothing to do with me, and that there was no way I could fix the situation. I politely ended the call. When I spoke to my associate later, I learned that the woman was his 82-year-old mother! She was filling in and answering the phones and was extremely stressed. This information made her behavior much more understandable. I was certainly glad that I had chosen to reframe the situation— for my sake and hers!

A woman in one of my classes was a supervisor for a group of receptionists. The receptionists were barraged daily with customer complaints. The supervisor advised that they look at each complaint as an opportunity to make a positive difference in someone's life. Another woman supervised a staff who answered the phones at a psychiatric hospital. The staff received many rude calls and were bothered by them. So the supervisor decided to start a contest. The person who received the rudest call of the week would win a prize. This brilliant bit of reframing transformed each nasty, stress-inducing call into an opportunity for fun. The staff was almost happy to get the rude calls. You can imagine them joyfully asking, "You called me a what? How do you spell that?" It didn't take much of a prize to help them gain some new perspective.

Some people get annoyed if they have to do some unexpected walking. They could reframe the situation and be thankful for the opportunity to get some exercise. There is nothing more ironic than people fighting to park as close as possible to the entrance of their health club so they can rush inside and work out on a treadmill.

❖ The Grocery Checkout Challenge

Imagine that you are in a grocery store. You pick the shortest checkout line because you are in a rush. However, as the line next to you moves like a greyhound, yours bogs down like a turtle in mud. You find yourself fuming that it is your fate to always pick the slowest line. You get annoyed as you watch the customer in front of you, who starts paying with a credit card but then changes his mind and decides that paying with a check would be better. Then he remembers the twelve coupons in his pocket. So the cashier starts over and the customer writes a new check. Your blood pressure continues to rise. How would you reframe this situation?

In these busy times, many of us rush from one task to another. We seldom have free time. I would reframe this wait at the grocery store as just that. I'd view it as an opportunity to focus on my breathing, reflect on my plans, maybe to list those aspects of my life for which I'm grateful. I might even chat with another person in line or indulge in the opportunity to flip through a magazine I wouldn't normally buy.

Free time! How many of us get enough? I know plenty of people who are stressed out over their lack of free time. Yet, ironically, in a typical week we find ourselves waiting through a variety of activities and getting stressed out about *that!* Whether you're put on hold while calling an office, standing in line at the Department of Motor Vehicles or at the bank, or stuck in a traffic jam, it is key to be able to reframe these waits as opportunities. Once you do this, potential times of stress become times to indulge yourself and relax.

⇨ *The Strong-Willed Child*

Few stages of life are more ripe for reframing exercises than early parenthood. Parenting has the potential to greatly increase our joy *and* our stress. For instance, most parents have experienced a child who is not cooperating and we feel like pulling our hair out.

In such a case, reframing offers the potential not just to reduce our stress load but to actually help the child as well. In his book *Setting Limits for Your Strong-Willed Child,* Robert MacKenzie reframes the situation by viewing a "stubborn" child as an "experiential learner." Some children have a strong desire to please and will quickly comply with requests. In contrast, the experiential learner needs to learn by experiencing a consequence. Remind yourself that your child is not acting stubborn because he is evil. He is probably acting that way because he gets away with it. As a bonus, he may get the opportunity to watch you act out your entertaining routine of yelling and negotiating. The consequences of his behavior have so far been fun for him. The first step is to set clear limits. Then, if he does not follow through, he gets the consequence (never physical punishment, however). For instance, you might say, "That whistle is too loud. If you blow it again inside the house, I will take it away." If your child blows it again, you calmly take the whistle away without the usual negotiations and extended warnings. In this way, the experiential learner eventually learns that your words have meaning. (The operative word, of course, is *eventually.*) Reframing your child from being stubborn (or worse) to being an "experiential learner" changes the emotional dynamics of the event and significantly reduces stress and worry.

Let's think about emotional and physical pain in another way. A weightlifter's muscles really hurt during and after a workout. If, out of the blue, your biceps started aching like that, you would knock on a doctor's door without delay. However, the weightlifter doesn't visit a doctor. She may even enjoy the pain. Why? To her, the pain has a meaning. It signifies that her muscles are growing and getting stronger. It reminds her that she's working hard. If the pain had no meaning, it would be something to be avoided. Child-birth is an example of intense pain that becomes part of a joyous experience because of its context: The pain is a necessary part of a wonderful event.

We have all gone through painful experiences, and when we can find meaning in those experiences, it helps to decrease our suffering. Perhaps you are distressed about your physical condition and don't like the way you look and feel. You can dwell on this distress, or you can use that feeling to motivate you to start an exercise program. Once you make that decision, it helps alleviate your suffering. The pain had a purpose. It was there not to make you miserable, but to stimulate you to take action and make changes.

Perhaps you suffer from a painful condition, such as rheumatoid arthritis. Even in this situation, you can choose to dwell on the stress and pain, or you can decide that your condition challenges you to find the best medical and behavioral treatments. Not only that, the pain might have further meaning if you start a support group to help others, or if you decide to help the local Arthritis Foundation. It may seem difficult, and pain is never fun, but the way you choose to view it can go a long way toward making it bearable.

Sally had an enlargement in her cheek that was thought to be a tumor. She was scheduled for an MRI scan and was terrified of the prospect of lying still in a tube for forty minutes while being scanned. She had worked herself into a frenzy and was about to ask her doctor for some Valium, when she decided to reframe the situation instead. She reminded herself that she was always busy, doing one thing or another. She never had time to sit and reflect about the things and people in her life for which she was grateful. The MRI scan could be a special time of solitude when no one would interrupt her. These thoughts gave a new meaning to the scan and soothed her anxiety. The tumor turned out to be benign. Since then, whenever Sally is in a traffic jam or similar circumstance, she reminds herself to appreciate her solitude and the opportunity to reflect on her life.

I would prefer it if neither my family nor I ever had any serious medical problems. However, my luck in that regard has not been perfect. Sooner or later, we all will see pain and illness in our families. It slightly decreases my pain to find meaning in the fact that any pain I have experienced increases my empathy for other people. It makes me a better physician, communicator, and human being. In this regard, I have learned more as a patient or a family member of a patient than I have in most of my medical school classes. I have also learned from other unfortunate events:

When our twins were eight months old, my wife and I planned a trip to visit relatives. About an hour into the trip, we had a blowout on the freeway. That's right, our right rear tire shredded with people going 70 miles an hour all around us. My wife very understandably said, "This is a nightmare!" It was a bad situation, but catastrophizing would not make it better. So I said, "This is definitely not ideal, but we'll manage." I was able to slowly drive onto the shoulder and get to a small road that was much less busy.

As my wife watched the boys, I emptied the back of the station wagon (which had been carefully packed to the brim) to get to the spare and then proceeded to change the tire. Together, my wife and I reframed the situation and agreed that it had been lucky that the flat had happened while we were together (as

opposed to her being alone with the boys); that it had happened
during the daytime; that it had not been raining; and that there
had been a small street just a half mile up the road where we
could much more safely stop than if we had been stuck on the
shoulder of the freeway.

If you are likely to encounter a particular stressful event, it may
help to use visualization to imagine yourself using the techniques
you have learned to effectively deal with the stress. The following
guided exercise is a good way to practice for such events.

⊙ Letting Go and Reframing Exercise. Disk 2, Track 3. Length: 10 Minutes

Play the assigned track. You will have the opportunity to explore
the use of mindfulness and reframing in dealing with several potentially stressful events. Find a quiet place to listen to the CD,
either lying down or sitting.

Are you having trouble figuring out a way to deal with or a new
way to look at a particular stressful situation? In *A Path with a
Heart,* Jack Kornfield describes a great visualization you can use
to help:

❖ Wise Visitor Visualization

Close your eyes and imagine you are in the midst of the situation.
Imagine the problem playing out the way it normally does, and
then at the peak of the stress, there is a knock at the door. When
you answer the door, you see the wisest, most compassionate person you can imagine. It could be a person you know personally, or

it could be a religious figure or prophet: Buddha, Jesus, Whoopi Goldberg—whomever you'd most like to see at that moment. That person offers to take over your body for a few minutes and handle the situation. Observe how he or she handles it. What can you learn? After she gives you back your body, imagine she gives you a piece of advice. What might she say? As you reflect on the advice, realize that it was you who had the wisdom and handled the situation all along.

Internal versus External Locus of Control

The best years of your life are the ones in which you decide your problems are your own. You do not blame them on your mother, the ecology or the president. You realize that you control your own destiny.

ALBERT ELLIS

Things turn out best for the people who make the best of the way things turn out.

JOHN WOODEN

Another important concept in cognitive therapy is *locus of control.* Having an "external locus of control" means thinking that your happiness and satisfaction depend primarily on the external environment. In contrast, having an "internal locus of control" means thinking that most of your happiness and satisfaction depend on the choices that you make and the way you view life. In short, do you look for your happiness from within or without? It's no surprise to learn that people with an internal locus of control tend to handle stress better than people with an external one. That's why one of the purposes of this book is to give you a more internal locus of control.

The self-help author Wayne Dyer tells a story of a visitor to a town asking one of the residents, "What is this town like?" "Well," the resident replied, "what was your old town like?" The visitor said, "People were angry, no one was nice, and it was not a very fun place at all." The resident said, "Well, our town is a lot like that."

A week later another visitor asked the same resident, "What is this town like?" The resident again asked, "What was your old town like?" The second visitor said, "In my old town, people were great. Everyone really looked out for their neighbors and cared about each other. It was a really pleasant place to live." The resident responded, "Our town is a lot like that." The way we view our circumstances has at least as much to do with our happiness as do the circumstances themselves.

The inspirational author W. Mitchell speaks throughout the world about how he has handled his unusual challenges. In the early 1970s, he had a severe burn accident affecting 65 percent of his body, including his face and hands. Just as his life was starting to go well again, he had a second accident, leaving him a paraplegic. At first, he found his wheelchair a prison, keeping him from doing the things he wanted to. Later, he reframed his situation, and the wheelchair became a magical apparatus that helped him travel throughout the world. He says that, before the accident, he "could do 9,000 things; after the accident 8,000 things." He chose to celebrate the 8,000 things he could do, rather than dwell on the 1,000 things he couldn't. His philosophy is embodied in the title of his wonderful book: *It's Not What Happens to You. It's What You Do about It.*

One of the things Mitchell's life story teaches us is that certain things that we say or think undermine our internal locus of control. Language—whether spoken by our lips or just echoing in our heads—can make a big difference. For instance, if I say, "He made me angry," I give all the responsibility for my anger to "him." I lose control over my own state of mind.

Think about these two phrases: (1) "I got angry because she left the top off the toothpaste." (2) "She left the top off the toothpaste and I got angry." In the first sentence, I had no choice but to be angry. That anger was the inevitable response to the action. The second sentence acknowledges that there were other options. There was still a connection between the action and the emotion, but the choice was mine. I could have thought it was funny and laughed. I could have been sad, or not cared. By restating the thought in a different way, I gave myself a choice in how I responded. This might sound insignificant, but the next time you think someone made you feel a certain way, try correcting yourself. You may be surprised by the subsequent change in your attitude.

We also limit ourselves with language in other ways. First thing one beautiful morning, when one of my sons was six years old, he spilled a drink. Then out of his mouth comes "I'm having a bad day." I had to chuckle (very quietly) to myself a little, since that phrase sounded a bit funny coming from a six-year-old. But how often, like my son, do we give ourselves self-fulfilling prophecies? One tiny thing goes wrong and Bam!—we think, "I'm having a bad day." And then, sure enough, we do have a bad day.

Consider the statements "I can't do math" and "Every time my boss criticizes me, I get very upset." Compare them with "In the past, I have had trouble with math" and "In the past, when my boss criticized me, I would get very upset." As you can see, the latter statements leave open your options for how to act in the future. They leave control, and responsibility, squarely on your shoulders. And just knowing that you have that internal locus of control goes a long way toward reducing stress and cultivating happiness.

Do you limit yourself with your thoughts in still other ways? Imagine a woman with four young children saying to herself, "I can't be happy in an unorganized house." With four young children, chances are that her house is disorganized much of the time. She has therefore limited herself to being unhappy much of the time. If you limit yourself to being happy only in very specific circumstances, you have lost a lot of potentially wonderful moments.

Developing an internal locus of control allows you to use yet another type of reframing. By now you have likely realized that the way you view a situation and the way you train your mind largely determine your stress level. Therefore, every hardship, every time you become irritated, can be seen as an opportunity to train your mind and to grow. Each challenge you meet makes you more prepared for the next one.

> Rosalyn had spent many hours while on vacation working on her first oil painting. Painting was a highlight of her trip, and she looked forward to hanging the framed artwork in her living room. Unfortunately, it was destroyed on the plane on the way home. Initially, she was understandably distressed.
>
> Rosalyn used several of the techniques described in this and the previous chapter to deal with her stress. She disputed irrational beliefs about the ruined artwork. Instead of "The vacation is ruined," she thought, "This is unfortunate." Instead of "How dumb of me not to get a box to protect the painting," she thought, "Now I know to protect my next painting with a box before I travel."
>
> She also reframed the situation. The most important part of this painting was the fun she had had working on it. She was now motivated to pursue a wonderful new hobby. That motivation was still unblemished.

Rosalyn also thought of Buddhist monks' spending several weeks making an intricate design out of sand. When the beautiful design is finished, it is appreciated. Then it is destroyed and the sand is poured into the ocean. The design is used as an example of life's impermanence. Rosalyn took a cue from the monks and used her disappointment as an opportunity to train her mind. By learning to deal with this situation effectively, she would be better prepared for life's future challenges. She would have honed her skills in disputing irrational beliefs, in reframing, and in letting go of thoughts of how life should be. Instead, she could enjoy life as it is—like the scenic drive at the end of the vacation.

Thoughts can unconsciously confine you to a certain view of reality. However, when you take a step back, you will recognize that the walls that formed that reality were just thoughts. Then you can renovate those mental walls into something more comfortable. You can see that, instead of being overwhelmed, you had a thought that you were overwhelmed. Instead of the traffic making you angry, you had a thought that the traffic made you angry. Taking this step back allows you to let certain thoughts go in order to enjoy the present moment. You may also dispute or reframe thoughts to better manage your stress.

Learning the ways in which we distort reality with our thoughts increases our insight, and disputing thoughts can be a useful tool. Most of the time, however, these processes aren't necessary. Just noticing the thought with mindfulness and letting it go are all that are needed. We need to take care not to ruminate—not to get caught in the trap of arguing with ourselves whether the thought is irrational or not. Either way, it is just a thought. And the only way to truly know reality is not to think about it, but to fully experience it as it is.

Additional Exercises

✎ List some examples of your irrational beliefs. Can you label what cognitive distortions they represent? How would you dispute these beliefs?

❖ Do you limit yourself by thinking you can be happy only if _____? Is this reality, or is it a choice you are imposing on yourself?

❖ Think back to a frustrating situation in your week. How could you have reframed it to change your stress response? How might the situation have played out differently if you had done so? If the situation is ongoing, what other element could you introduce—like the prize for the rudest call that the supervisor offered—to change the dynamics?

7

Slow Down

Half our life is spent trying to find something to do with the time
we have rushed through life trying to save.

WILL ROGERS

For fast-acting relief, try slowing down.

LILY TOMLIN

ACCORDING TO A popular story, two cardiologists, Meyer Friedman and Ray H. Rosenman, pondered the rapid rate at which
their waiting-room chairs were wearing out. Looking into the
room, they noticed a very impatient, anxious group of patients sitting almost on the front edges of their chairs. This observation
gave them the idea that a certain personality style is associated
with a higher risk of heart disease. They labeled this personality
style "type A." Following this observation, the two cardiologists,
along with biochemist Sanford O. Byers, began exploring the relationship of personality style and heart disease. Several studies
did indeed show a connection between type A personality and
heart disease.

People with type A personalities continuously struggle to accomplish more and more. Type B personalities tend to be more

mellow and laid back. With the type A personality, there is a sense of time urgency, often when there is no real reason to rush. The urgency includes: talking very quickly and finishing others' sentences, driving and eating fast, and multitasking.

Type A people tend to be more aggressive and hostile. Although there has been some recent controversy about the effect of type A behavior on heart disease, excessive anger and hostility have been clearly shown to be related to heart disease in several studies. One study followed 1,305 men for seven years. The men with the greatest levels of anger had 2.66 times the risk of developing a heart problem. Additionally, time urgency, impatience, and hostility are associated with a significant increase in the long-term risk of high blood pressure.

The type A personality can be changed. The aggravation, impatience, anger, and irritation associated with this personality style do not usually produce good results at work or at home. The researchers advise people with type A personalities to take time with friends, avoid interrupting people, practice waiting in line and driving in the slow lane, and practice eating slowly and fully tasting their food.

There are many other ways to integrate relaxation into your life. The therapeutic benefit of owning a pet is becoming increasingly recognized. In fact, "pet therapy" is becoming popular in hospitals and nursing homes around the country. We are likely to get even more benefit from the love we give a pet than from the love we receive from the pet.

Other advice includes learning to empathize with others; taking time for cultural activities such as museums, art, and music; and avoiding trying to do many tasks at once. (Perhaps it is reasonable at work to dictate or write a "to-do list" while you are sitting on hold for 10 minutes. This is still, in a sense, doing one thing at a time. However, when I found myself dialing a phone, dictating as

I waited for someone to answer, and then forgetting whom I had called—well, that was too much!)

If you rush through the workday at a harried pace, interrupting people and trying to do several projects at once, just to get home thirty minutes earlier, it probably is not worth the additional stress. Although it is important to have time at home, it is better to enjoy working an 8½-hour day than to spend an 8-hour day in distress. People with a type A personality often worry about wasting time, so I found this quotation from a lecture by researcher Diane Ulmer particularly relevant: "A day wasted by not enjoying it is the real waste of time." In fact, I might add that a *moment* wasted by not enjoying it is the real waste of time.

Enjoy the little things, for one day
You may look back and realize they
Were the big things.

ROBERT BRAULT

Ulmer feels that the major factor in the development of the type A personality style is low self-esteem and a continuing need to prove oneself. Low self-esteem cannot be improved by the frantic pursuit of material objects or achievements. It is important to have an inherent sense of self-worth. Most people in my classes say that they are willing to believe that all of us have inherent worth, independent of any accomplishments. If you have a thought otherwise, remember it is just a thought that can be let go, and then you can return to enjoy the next breath. If it surfaces again, you gently let it go again.

No one can make you feel inferior without your consent.

ELEANOR ROOSEVELT

It may even be worthwhile to ponder who you really are. As your mind is still and you gaze at a sunset or smell a rose, you can ask, "Am I just this body? Am I just this personality? Am I just my thoughts? Indeed, who watches my thoughts? Am I really something much more?"

Sometimes rushing not only increases our stress but also really does not save any time at all.

Cindy worked in a retail store. Like many people in the retail business, she was often rushed for time. One day, a demanding customer was taking a long time at the store. Instead of spending an extra two minutes addressing this person's concerns, Cindy became impatient. By cutting her time with this customer short, she saved those two minutes. However, later that day she remembered what she'd done and it bothered her. She spent some time justifying her actions to herself, then spent some more time feeling bad and wondering if she had been rude.

The next day, the customer complained to Cindy's supervisor. Cindy then had to spend an extra 30 minutes writing a response to his complaint. Cindy might not have done anything technically wrong, but in the long run she saved only two minutes by rushing a conversation with the customer, and those two minutes ultimately cost her much more time feeling stressed about the interaction and responding to the complaint.

The book *The House of God* is a sarcastic novel that looks at the difficult life of medical residents. In the book, experienced residents teach new residents certain "laws" of residency. One of the laws has to do with how one should act in dealing with a cardiac arrest (when a patient's heart stops): "At a cardiac arrest, the first procedure is to take your own pulse." For some-one who has never "run a code" (i.e., directed the staff in car-ing for someone having a cardiac arrest), this law probably seems like a joke in poor taste. Only those of us who have run a code understand it.

When someone's heart has stopped, there is the temptation to frantically try to do something. However, when you are frantic in a code, you are inefficient and more likely to make a mistake. Even when someone's heart stops, it can be much more effective for a doctor to take two or three seconds and one diaphragmatic breath before acting. That way, the doctor can remember her or his training and act efficiently and thoughtfully. I would not actu-ally take my own pulse. A one-minute delay is a bad idea. But a couple of seconds to take that diaphragmatic breath could help save a life.

I know that most of you aren't in the position of having to re-spond to cardiac arrests. But consider this: Not many emergen-cies are more pressing than someone's heart stopping; yet, even then, it makes sense to take one diaphragmatic breath before act-ing. If you need to push someone off the train tracks before a train hits him, you might not have those two seconds. For almost all of your other "personal emergencies," you can and should spare at least that amount of time.

In our frantic lives, we sometimes have to remind ourselves that we're not in the middle of an emergency. Several years ago, I occasionally worked weekend shifts as a doctor in an un-derstaffed urgent-care center. Since there were no scheduled appointments, patient waiting times were often long. One Sun-day, an unusually large number of patients had to be seen, and the wait was well over two hours. I found myself exhibiting type

A behavior—frequently interrupting patients and rushing them along. Suddenly I realized that no one was dying.

I decided that, on Monday, I would advise the administration that we needed more staff on weekends in the future. But in the meantime, I needed a strategy for the current weekend. My type A strategy of rushing and interrupting patients was saving only a few minutes, at best. And it was unfair to the patients. If someone had already waited two hours, the last thing he or she needed was a doctor who interrupted every other sentence.

Instead, I decided to shift my perspective and give each patient a more considered interaction with me. Seeing a doctor who listened empathetically would certainly be worth an additional 10-minute wait to these patients. On that long day, I saw over 40 patients. However, I was not stressed, and the patients did seem more appreciative, despite their wait, since their problems were carefully and considerately addressed.

When Do I Rush?

Are there times when you typically rush unnecessarily? List some of these times. Then consider solutions. Should you wake up a little earlier so you don't have to rush? Are you overscheduled? Or can you just practice taking your time without any of these external changes?

1. _____

2. _____

3. _____

4. _____

5. _____

⇨ Slow-Motion Living

On occasion, when you have a little more time, try setting aside that time to practice moving very slowly. Do a walking meditation, and bring your awareness to the sensations in your legs and feet. As you reach to open a door, notice your arm reaching. You might even note to yourself, "Reaching." As you turn the doorknob, notice your hand turning the doorknob. Of course, it is not practical to always move this slowly. Perhaps, for the few minutes after a sitting meditation, you can try moving slowly and mindfully. If you are going on vacation or retreat, maybe you can spend more time moving at a slow, purposeful pace. Practicing this type of mindfulness in slow motion can carry over as you resume a more normal pace.

8

Keep Life in Perspective

Rule #1: Don't sweat the small stuff. Rule #2: It's all small stuff.

ROBERT ELIOT

As a doctor, I get to see a variety of faces of humanity—one right after another. I get to ponder questions like "How can one person be dying of pancreatic cancer and be doing well emotionally, while another person is stressed out beyond belief by having one room in his mansion remodeled?" I've learned that one of the more important ways to cope with stress is to learn how to keep one's problems in perspective.

One day a student became very upset, so he went to speak with his teacher. The teacher asked him, "If you had a billion dollars and you lost five dollars, would you be upset?" The student said, "Of course not." The teacher then said to the student, "You are a billionaire." The student then understood that when he considered all he had to be thankful for—his family, friends, and health—he was, in a sense, a billionaire. The next time something went wrong, he thought to himself, "Five bucks," and smiled.

⇨ Five-Bucks Reminder

In most instances, if we can take a step back and put a problem in perspective, our stress level decreases markedly. The next time something happens that distresses you, say to yourself, "Five bucks," and remind yourself that you are a billionaire.

Gratitude

There are only two ways to live your life—one is as if everything is a miracle, the other is as though nothing is a miracle.

ALBERT EINSTEIN

We can only be said to be alive in those moments when our hearts are conscious of our treasures.

THORNTON WILDER

One of the most effective ways to keep problems in perspective is to remember to appreciate what we have. Often, we ignore many of the important things in life for which we could be grateful, partly because our brains cannot focus on too much information at once. If we are in a room illuminated by fluorescent lights, after a while we no longer hear the hum of the lights. If we are at a dinner party with four simultaneous conversations going on and we focus on one conversation, we do not hear the others. Our brains can process only a very small percentage of the information gathered by our senses at any one time. Right now, are you focused on your right big toe? Prior to my mentioning it, my guess is probably not. Unless your toe is hurting, you were probably totally unaware of it. Yet, if you choose to, you can focus on your right big toe. You can also choose to focus on the hum of the fluorescent lights. Our brains are constantly bombarded by sensory input from all five of our senses. It follows that, at any given time, our brains can focus on only a relatively small amount of the information gathered by our senses. If we consider all the memories, plans, and other information that our brains contain, it becomes obvious that we can focus on only a minute fraction of our brain's content at any one particular time. We can use this quality of our brains to our advantage by choosing what we want to focus on.

Often, it is helpful to remind ourselves of what we have to be grateful for throughout the day. You can contemplate this subject whenever you are feeling down or stressed. You can also make it a regular part of your day (at the end of your meditation or another time).

Imagine the most awe-inspiring scenic view that you have ever seen. Recently, I was at a restaurant that had such a view. On three sides of the restaurant were breathtaking vistas of the Pacific Ocean. When the waiter was asked what it was like to work in that environment, he said that, most of the time, he forgot about the view. Only occasionally would he remind himself to appreciate the scenery.

We have grown accustomed to many positive aspects of our lives. Like that waiter, we need to remind ourselves to appreciate our blessings. List the things in your life for which you are grateful: your health, the people in your life, and even a warm shower. Be grateful that you have food to eat. If you can see, be grateful for your vision; if you cannot see, be grateful for your hearing. If you have trouble hearing, be grateful for your senses of touch and taste.

If only people who worry about their liabilities would think about the riches they do possess, they would stop worrying. Would you sell both your eyes for a million dollars . . . or your two legs . . . or your hands . . . or your hearing? Add up what you do have, and you'll find that you won't sell them for all the gold in the world. The best things in life are yours, if you can appreciate yourself.

DALE CARNEGIE

When we respond to the challenges life hands us, we can find positive aspects of unfortunate situations. Helen Keller wrote, "I thank God for my handicaps, for through them, I have found myself, my work, and my God." Our culture tends to be preoccupied with looks. Golda Meir said, "Not being beautiful was the true blessing. . . . Not being beautiful forced me to develop my inner resources. The pretty girl has a handicap to overcome."

In her book *Simple Abundance,* Sarah Ban Brethnach strongly recommends making a "gratitude journal." At the end of the day, you write down five things for which you are grateful. Some days it may be something small, like the new birdhouse you bought; other days, you might list more serious items, such as health and family. You might review yesterday's five items in the morning. Before you know it, you will have a whole book full of items for which you can be grateful. You can refer to that book whenever you want to.

✐ Gratitude Journal

Start your own gratitude journal. Take a moment to list some of the people and parts of your life for which you are grateful. At a bare minimum, fill in the spaces below now. Even better, get a separate journal or notebook that you can fill up and refer to on a daily basis. During difficult times, it's important to refer to this list or to add to it.

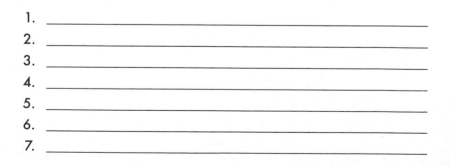

1. _____
2. _____
3. _____
4. _____
5. _____
6. _____
7. _____

8. _____
9. _____
10. _____
11. _____
12. _____
13. _____
14. _____
15. _____
16. _____
17. _____
18. _____
19. _____
20. _____

⇨ Gratitude Practice

To experience how a sense of gratitude can positively affect your life, try the following experiment. Several times an hour, over the course of a day, look for something for which to be grateful and actually make one of the following statements to yourself:

○ "I am grateful to have (blank)."
○ "I feel privileged to have (blank) in my life."
○ "I am so lucky to have (blank)."
○ Or pray, "Thank you for (blank)."

Make these statements with feeling. As you say how grateful you are for a friend or family member in your life, visualize his or her face. Think of different special moments. Think of your health, your ability to see, hear, and/or feel beauty. Being thankful for the food on your plate (and even the ability to smell and taste good food) will also enhance your mindfulness.

During the day that you purposefully repeat those statements to yourself, notice how you feel. Making this a regular practice will make a very positive difference in your life.

Purpose and Altruism

Dennis was a 65-year-old gentleman who had been retired for 10 years when he came to see me. About 20 years prior to the visit, Dennis had had a back injury. Most of Dennis's stress revolved around his chronic back pain. Since that time, he had tried multiple pain medications, had attempted physical therapy several times, and had gone through two back surgeries. He had also participated in an intensive, six-month pain management program with no success. His pain was managed only by huge daily doses of morphine.

On one visit, Dennis shared with me that his need for the pain medication had decreased dramatically. He rarely used his morphine. He felt incredibly well and, most days, did not need any pain medicine at all. To what did Dennis attribute this remarkable change?

Dennis had started a job in which he sold equipment to disabled people. Not only did he really enjoy the job, but he also truly felt that he was making a positive difference in many people's lives. He felt wonderful and had had at least a 90 percent improvement in both his pain and his stress.

After Victor Frankl survived the horrors of a Nazi concentration camp during World War II, he realized that most of the survivors had one trait in common: a strong sense of purpose. Perhaps it was a book that they knew only they could write, or they needed to stay alive for a family member, or, as in his case, they needed to stay alive to tell the story of the holocaust, so that hopefully it would never occur again. This strong sense of purpose had helped keep these survivors alive and had helped them put up with the horrible conditions in the concentration camps.

All of us can gain perspective in our lives by developing a sense of purpose and a sense of making a positive impact in others' lives. Choose a job, hobby, or volunteer work for which you can have a passion, and that makes a contribution to the lives of others. Anne Frank said, "How wonderful it is that nobody need wait a single moment before starting to improve the world."

Whatever work you do, do it with integrity and in a way that contributes to others. Helping others shows you what is important and quiets your mind from its preoccupation with complaints about relatively small problems. The writer William Bennet said, "There are no menial jobs, only menial attitudes." You can be bored as you sell flowers at a flower stand, or you can seek to make each person you deal with a little happier. Since flowers are often given as presents, you can acknowledge that you are indirectly bringing beauty to people you might never meet. You can struggle working in construction, or you can take pride in acquiring skills and building useful and well-made structures.

There is a classic story about three brick masons working on the same job. When asked about his job, the first said, "I have this boring job of placing one brick after another. It is boring, lowly, and demeaning." A second mason said about his job, "The work is solid and it allows me to provide for my family." When the third mason was asked about his job, he said, "I'm building a cathedral that will last for hundreds and maybe even thousands of years. It will offer both physical shelter and spiritual comfort to unknown multitudes. I do my work carefully because I am so privileged to be a part of this great project."

If you seek happiness for yourself, you can have everything in the world and still be unhappy. But, if you seek happiness for others, you'll find happiness yourself. That's the way it is.

TRULSHIG RINCHOPE

Is the above quotation true, or does it just sound nice? There are many unhappy rich people. The gossip magazines are filled with their stories. The most fulfilled people have learned the joy of true compassion. Caring for others decreases our inner chatter about what we "lack." It provides us a stronger sense of purpose and helps us put our lives in perspective. It lets us experience the joy of contributing and compassion.

I don't know what your destiny will be, but one thing I know: the only ones among you who will be truly happy are those who will have sought and found how to serve.

ALBERT SCHWEITZER

This is the true joy in life, the being used for a purpose recognized by yourself as a mighty one; the being thoroughly worn out before you are thrown on the scrap heap; the being a force of nature instead of a feverish selfish little clod of ailments and grievances complaining that the world will not devote itself to making you happy.

GEORGE BERNARD SHAW

From what we get, we can make a living: what we give, however, makes a life.

ARTHUR ASHE

The research confirms that altruism is associated with health. For instance, epidemiologist James House studied 2,700 men in Tecumsah, Michigan. Men who did not do volunteer work were two-and-a-half times more likely to die during the study period than men who volunteered at least once a week.

Altruism can take many forms. You can help others in small, everyday ways or take on much more ambitious projects. In his book *Illusions,* Richard Bach wrote, "Here is a test to find whether your mission on Earth is finished: if you're alive, it isn't."

It is worthwhile to take a moment to reflect on what activities you feel naturally passionate about. Incorporating those things into your work or other parts of your life can help bring perspective and joy.

How can we not feel overwhelmed by all the suffering in the world? This question brings us back to mindfulness. As we hear of another's suffering, sadness is natural. Instead of pushing away the sadness, just notice it and feel its intensity. From being present with this sadness, compassion arises. Action then naturally flows from the compassion. Instead of acting out of guilt, we act out of this compassion. If all the problems in the world seem overwhelming, we keep in mind what Mother Teresa said: "If you can't feed a hundred people, then just feed one."

Acting naturally out of compassion brings a deep contentment and connection. It is wonderful to have lofty goals. However, stay focused on the action in front of you. If one is too attached to the final result, it is easy to get discouraged. Instead, mindfully take joy in each small act, and amazing things will be accomplished.

Also keep in mind that as we take care of others, we need to care for ourselves. If we spend no time rejuvenating ourselves with exercise, hobbies, and friendships, we will find it harder to give joyfully. I e-mailed a work associate about my surprise that she had responded to a work e-mail on a Sunday night. Her entire e-mail response was "24/7/365." This response is similar to the story I not infrequently hear from caregivers of disabled spouses: They give care 24 hours a day, 7 days a week, and 365 days a year. We all need a little time off from caring for others in order to care for ourselves. I encourage caregivers to seek help from family, friends, adult day-care centers, organizations like the Alzheimer's Association, and so on. How can one give water from a well that is never refilled? We will speak of this topic more in the next chapter.

✎ Giving Back

List additional ways that you might contribute to your society (large or small).

1. _____
2. _____
3. _____
4. _____

✎ Making a Difference

Use this next list to remind yourself of how your current job, hobbies, and family life make a difference to those around you. List the activities, and also list how they make a positive difference to others.

Activity	How the activity helps others

Humor

Laughter is a form of internal jogging. It moves your organs around. It enhances respiration. It is an igniter of great expectations.

NORMAN COUSINS

Another way to gain perspective is through a sense of humor. Our sense of humor can help carry us through those times that might otherwise be much more difficult. Develop your sense of humor by watching funny movies, reading the comics and humorous books, or searching for new jokes on the Internet. You might even want to practice telling jokes, so you can make others laugh.

Humor can often be found in stressful situations. How might we use humor to defuse a potentially stressful situation? Joel Goodman, director of the Humor Project in Saratoga Springs, New York, recommends that you imagine how your favorite comedian would react in a similar scenario. When one thing after another goes wrong, it's easy to become frustrated. Sometimes frustration can be turned around if you throw a little humor in.

Once I was traveling to give a lecture. The plane was late, and everyone else's luggage came off before ours. Somewhere across town, there were several hundred people in a rented hall waiting for me to give a talk—perhaps on the importance of being on time—and it was getting later and later. Finally our luggage started to arrive. . . . One suitcase had sprung open, and clothes were spread all over the conveyer belt. Another piece of luggage was obviously damaged. The people traveling with me were more and more upset. Finally I said, "Relax, this is funny. In a few weeks we'll be telling stories about tonight and laughing about it. If it'll be funny then it's funny now." And we started looking at the situation as if it were a Woody Allen movie. When some of the luggage didn't arrive, we smiled. When the car rental company didn't have our reservation (or cars), we laughed. When we heard there was a taxi strike, we howled.

JOHN-ROGER WILLIAMS

In one moment, the tears might be flowing like Niagara Falls or we might be shaking with stress like a bowl of gelatin in an earthquake. Then, suddenly, by seeing the humor in the situation, we can laugh. Remember, if it will be funny in 10 years, it's funny now.

People were very stressed at Sally's workplace. It seemed that much of the staff was on vacation in August. The remaining staff was therefore getting behind in processing orders. As they got further behind, they had to respond to more and more phone calls about the late orders. These further delayed the process. Several hour-long and seemingly irrelevant work meetings made the situation worse. Sally designed a sign for the bulletin board that said, "Seven-hour meeting today to discuss why the work is backlogged." The humor seemed to draw the staff together and lighten the mood, though Sally is currently unemployed (just joking!).

It is essential to learn to laugh at yourself. Learn to laugh at your occasional neurotic behavior and perceived shortcomings.

Accurate Assessments

In order to make decisions and judgments, we need to assess risk. Occasionally, we may increase our stress by miscalculating risks. For instance, we may get extremely stressed on an airplane although the risk of dying may be far greater on your daily car commute. We tend to react to what has been sensationalized in the media. There is no way to decrease your risks in life to zero. Therefore, it is essential to pay attention to what the real risks are and not to overreact to what the media have sensationalized. Driving carefully and using a seat belt will decrease your risk much more than fantasizing what might happen on your plane trip.

Another place where accurate assessments are helpful is in determining what is required by a particular job. Perfectionism can definitely increase one's level of stress. Additionally, when we feel compelled to do everything perfectly, we may actually be less productive at work. It is essential to learn to prioritize. If we spend an hour writing a "perfect" short e-mail to an associate, we have less time to accomplish other work. It is admirable to want to excel, but it's important not to devote so much time and attention to a single tree that the forest dies of inattention. If we spend more time and effort than is warranted on a particular job, other parts of our work or family life will likely suffer.

Your Perfectionist Streak

List three times you have displayed an undue amount of perfectionism. How might you change to be more productive and relaxed?

1. _____
2. _____
3. _____

When we are stressed about a given situation, it may help to accurately assess what would happen if the outcome is unfavorable. In other words, we may ask, "What's the worst that will happen?" Often, we find that answering that question decreases our panic. We may be acting as if something is a life-or-death matter when, in fact, nothing drastic will happen if the situation does not work out. There are no cookie-cutter answers to assessing risk, assessing the amount of effort a particular job requires, and assessing "What's the worst that will happen?" However, just asking those questions can be very useful.

Tony's job was much more difficult because many of his coworkers had been laid off. Complicating matters, his new manager was rude and had unrealistic expectations. The manager expected Tony to take on what had previously been the responsibility of three people. Not only was Tony anxious most of the day at work, but his home life was also suffering. I empathized with Tony's difficult situation. Then I asked, "If you spoke with your boss about the problem, what is the worst that would happen?" Tony realized that if he was assertive and politely stood up to his boss, either his work life would improve or he might get fired from a job that he hated. He did not like the idea of getting fired, but if he did, he would collect unemployment as he looked for a better job. Either outcome was better than what he was already enduring. Knowing that, he felt less stress and decided to stand up for himself.

Things Change

There is one constant principle in the universe and that is "Things change." Time does not stand still. Life constantly changes. When people are depressed, they sometimes think the situation will never change and the depression will last forever. However, you may rest assured during the hardest times that, as the saying goes, "This, too, shall pass."

It is comforting to remember that life's difficulties often eventually work out, one way or another. We often hear, "When one door closes, another opens." But as Helen Keller observed, "When one door closes, another opens; but often we look so long at the closed door that we do not see the one which has opened for us." We have all been upset over a particular event and then later realized that it was actually good fortune in disguise. Not infrequently, I have heard of someone's being laid off from a job only to eventually find a job that was much better.

What the caterpillar calls the end of the world, the master calls a butterfly.

RICHARD BACH

My father-in-law was moving from Northern to Southern California. He rented a truck and a trailer. Just as he was ready to leave, he found that the trailer was incompatible with the truck. As a result, the brake lights wouldn't work. He was forced to leave the trailer in Northern California, knowing that he would need to drive an extra 12 hours round-trip to retrieve it. You can imagine that he might be thinking, "What a catastrophe!" As he set out without the trailer, the truck had a tire blowout. He pulled to the side of the road easily. He later learned that, if he had had a blowout while driving with the trailer, his truck would likely have jackknifed, and he could have been in a very serious accident. This seeming "catastrophe" of an incompatible trailer might have saved his life.

Sometimes, a children's story has an important message for adults. In *It Could Have Been Worse*, a young mouse becomes upset on several occasions as he trips or falls down. He has one "mishap" after another, so he thinks he is having a terrible day. However, he never seems to notice that each time he falls, it helps him narrowly miss being caught by one of several predators. Each time, he is slightly bruised, but still alive. This story shows children (and their parents) that what seems like an unfortunate event on the surface may, in reality, be a truly fortunate one. Sometimes, we, like the mouse, are not aware of the whole story.

Many religions teach that when circumstances do not look good on the surface, we must trust that there is a larger plan. Having this view helps people cope with disappointment and also decreases worry by increasing confidence that they can handle whatever the future brings. Some people may put this trust in God, and others may trust their own ability to deal with whatever "comes down the pike." Either way, this type of trust can be tremendously comforting in times of potential stress.

I asked God for strength, that I might achieve;
I was made weak, that I might learn humbly to obey.
I asked for health, that I might do greater things;
I was given infirmity, that I might do better things.
I asked for riches, that I might be happy;
I was given poverty, that I might be wise.
I asked for power, that I might have the praise of men;
I was given weakness, that I might feel the need of God.
I asked for all things, that I might enjoy life;
I was given life, that I might enjoy all things.
I received nothing that I asked for, but everything I had hoped for.
Almost despite myself, my unspoken prayers were answered.
I am, among all people, most richly blessed.

ANONYMOUS

Sally told me that, as a young mother, she was overwhelmed with stress. Her young son had been diagnosed with diabetes. This diagnosis required extra care and contributed to extra worry in her already busy life. She was having trouble functioning day to day.

Finally, she said, she "gave the problem to God." What I think she meant by that was that she decided to trust that God would help to take care of the situation in one way or another. The solution would all be part of God's plan. Sally worked just as hard providing care to her son, but it was done with less stress. When Sally started to feel too stressed, she would tell herself that she was "giving her problem to God," and she would feel a tremendous sense of relief.

In the midst of a longer meditation, sometimes I pretend that there are only a few moments of the meditation left. In that way, I savor every breath. In the same way, as I realize how short our lives are, I treasure each moment.

The ultimate way to gain perspective may be to remind ourselves that our time on earth is limited. Do not waste time complaining about the "small stuff." Instead, enjoy the ride, including all of the bumps and curves in the road.

It's only when we truly know and understand that we have a limited time on earth—and that we have no way of knowing when our time is up—that we will begin to live each day to the fullest, as if it was the only one we had.

ELISABETH KÜBLER-ROSS

It's easy to think of the phrase "Live each day as you would your last" as a worn cliché. How can we make this saying more helpful? How can we really put it to use?

⇨ *Your Last Moments on Earth*

Whatever you do next, pretend you only have a few moments to live. When you pretend there is time only for this last activity, what is that hug like? What is that bite of food like? What is that shower like? What is that kiss like? What is that conversation like? Don't just read this; really try it with your next activity. Notice the level of mindfulness you have. Notice how you relish that activity. Don't pretend it is your last day; pretend these are your last moments. See how you treasure them. See how you can luxuriate in the moment—how you savor just this step, this breath.

Let's end this section with a tad more reflection about things changing. When one says, "This too shall pass," it often is interpreted as: "Grin and bear it for now, since it will get better"— almost like life is a big kidney stone, and you can barely wait for it to pass. There is a more productive way to hold life's changes: Marvel at how this very moment is unique—never to happen again. Turn your head just a few degrees and notice how the sights change. Everything: physical sensations, emotions, thoughts, tastes, touch, fragrances—all are in a constant state of flux.

Often, we are surprised by change. When we mindfully observe the arising and passing of each sensation, thought, and emotion, amazing insights occur. When we see change over and over again, in every moment of life, we are less surprised by it. We know it is inevitable and we can "enjoy the ride." When you have spent time noticing that all things change, the car breaking down is not the end of the world—it's expected. Cars do not last forever—nothing does. By being aware of the arising and passing of all we encounter, we enhance our ability to be mindful and decrease our stress over life's inevitable changes.

⇨ *Meditation on Arising and Passing*

Experiment with the mantra "arising" (as you inhale) and "passing" (as you exhale). Marvel at the uniqueness of this moment.

Spend some time paying attention to how sensations, thoughts, and emotions change. With your eyes open turn your head and watch the visual changes. Notice changes as you breathe, changes as you move, changes in sound, and so on. Mindfully pay attention to the arising and passing of all phenomena.

✐List several specific ways to keep your life in perspective:

9

Improve Your Lifestyle

At the end of your life, you will never regret not having passed one more test, not winning one more verdict, or not closing one more deal. You will regret time not spent with a husband, a friend, a child, or a parent.

BARBARA BUSH

Balance

One of the keys and challenges to a healthy lifestyle is to balance all of the different areas of your life. When you take time to develop multiple aspects of your life, including relationships, family, work, and hobbies, any single problem can seem less stressful. In other words, you do not have "all of your eggs in one basket." If your boss yells at you, you can still get satisfaction from your friends, family, and/or hobbies.

There is no better time to find balance in your life than the present. Not infrequently, I see patients with two children working stressful 70-hour weeks. As we contemplate the past 10 or 20 years of our lives, we might be surprised at how quickly the time went. As we get older, the time seems to go faster and faster. I have not heard anyone on his or her deathbed say that he or she wished to have spent more time working. If you don't take the time to enjoy life now, when are you going to do it?

Maintaining balance in our lives sometimes requires us to resist our cultural preoccupation with money and possessions. We are continually bombarded by advertisements telling us what we need to purchase to be happy. Once our basic needs are met, most material objects bring, at best, very brief happiness. We would be much happier if we learned that we do not need most of what the advertisers say we need. Most of us know rich people who are unhappy. If we do not know them personally, we hear of wealthy celebrities who suffer from depression and even commit suicide. On the other hand, many people of much more modest means thoroughly enjoy life. Too often, we find ourselves in extra financial stress, since we have been sold on the idea that we need that extra-fancy car or expensive clothes. Then we must work many more hours, possibly at multiple jobs, to meet expenses.

Simplifying your life can often reduce stress. For instance, you might find that you are better off with a smaller house that is easier to maintain and has a smaller mortgage. This smaller house might allow you to work less and spend more time with your family, friends, and hobbies. Another way to simplify your life is by giving away or selling old objects that are never used (after consulting with your spouse and family, of course; let's not start any huge fights).

Involve the whole family. Teach your children the importance of charity. Will they help by giving away their old unused toys? If your children are too young to appreciate the logic of giving away their old toys, there is another option. Have them take their old toys to a used-toy store. They can go in with a bunch of old toys and get a few dollars to buy a small new toy.

Who is rich? He that rejoices in his portion.

BENJAMIN FRANKLIN

The trouble with the rat race is that, even if you win, you're still a rat.

LILY TOMLIN

Bonnie's parents were well off financially, and she had become accustomed to a relatively costly lifestyle growing up. She and her husband worked hard to continue that lifestyle, and before she knew it, she was working four jobs. Although none of the jobs were full time, the combination was much more than full time. After taking my stress management class, she started to realize that her lifestyle was costing her more than just money. Her stress was markedly reduced when she made some changes, including selling her expensive car and quitting two of her jobs.

One way to improve the balance of your life is to set aside time away from work in order to have time focused on family, friends, and/or spirituality. Many religions recommend a Sabbath day. When we are younger, we sometimes do not see the wisdom of traditions. As we gain more experience, it may make a lot more sense to make sure that at least one day is set aside for activities other than work. At least one day a week and at least some time each day away from work will help keep our lives more fulfilled and balanced.

Balance is important not only between work and family life, but also between different parts of family life. A good friend told me that she and her husband had some marital tension. She wondered whether counseling would be a good idea. Her husband suggested that, instead of spending money on a counselor, they spend money on a babysitter for a date night once a week. Counselors help many people learn to communicate better. However, this couple was communicating fairly well. They just needed some time devoted to their marriage, as opposed to having all of their energies spent just on work and children.

Balance is important between all of the aspects of our lives, including work, marriage, children, relaxation, hobby, and exercise. Stop competing with others, trying to show how much stress you can tolerate. Instead, create a life in which you take pride in your balanced, healthy lifestyle.

⇨ *Day of Mindfulness*

Consider taking an occasional day or half day off to devote to mindfulness. You can incorporate different forms of sitting meditation, walking meditation, and yoga. If possible, spend some time in a natural setting.

Time Management

Why should we be in such desperate haste to succeed, and in such desperate enterprises? If a man does not keep pace with his companions, perhaps it is because he hears a different drummer.

HENRY DAVID THOREAU

Simplifying your life also involves time management. Many attempt to pack their schedules tighter than a rhinoceros in a spandex jumpsuit. If you have an 11 a.m. appointment, you might find yourself trying to do six errands before the appointment. It is best to adjust your schedule so you're not stressed by constantly rushing or running late. Plan to do just the two or three most important errands before the appointment, and make a more realistic schedule for the other errands.

If you were flying across country, would you leave only 10 minutes for a connection between two flights? Not unless you can run a 100-yard dash in five seconds while carrying your luggage in your teeth. You need to leave a little margin in case the first flight is a little late or the gates aren't right next to each other. If you try to continually run your life at maximum capacity, without leaving any room for unexpected occurrences, or even room to relax once in a while, you will burn out. In other words, avoid scheduling yourself at 100 percent capacity. Our technological progress was supposed to give us all sorts of free time; instead, we are working more and have less free time than our ancestors. Also, workers in the U.S. tend to work longer hours than those in many other countries. Therefore, compared to the rest of history and with other countries, this current cultural norm is not normal at all. We, as a culture, are out of sorts with what is healthy. Scheduling a little margin between your activities will markedly decrease your stress.

Although there are many benefits to technology, technology itself often intrudes on our leisure. There used to be times when we were not reachable. Then came home and work telephones. They were intrusive enough. Now our bosses, families, friends, and even strangers can call our cell phones, thus interrupting us at almost any time and in almost any place. If we do not answer our cell phones, we might be paged. As if e-mail were not intrusive enough, along came the invention of instant messaging: "Respond now . . . I know you are on the computer."

You have a choice. Technology can be a tool or it can be a master. Knowing when to turn off your cell phone is a skill worth developing. Even if a phone is on, it does not always have to be answered. Signing up for the telemarketing "do not call" list can decrease nuisance calls (www.donotcall.gov). If you use your computer's instant messaging, know when to turn it off. You do not have to reply to or even read each e-mail as soon as it is received. Is it more efficient to set aside a certain time to work on the e-mails?

Routing your e-mail through a service with a good spam filter can also help with your efficiency.

While we are on the subject of computers and technology, it is worth emphasizing that an ounce of prevention is worth a pound of cure. Some things are learned the hard way. From experience, I know it is worthwhile to have a good backup system for my computer. With inexpensive external hard drives and even off-site backup services available, there are fewer excuses for not appropriately backing up information.

In *Don't Sweat the Small Stuff with Your Family,* Richard Carlson describes the maintenance of the Golden Gate Bridge. He states that "the bridge is painted almost every day of the year." In other words, as soon as they finish painting the bridge, they need to start all over again. Carlson compares this routine to the maintenance of a house. There is always something that could be done. In fact, many areas of our lives are similar to painting the Golden Gate Bridge. We can decrease our stress by realizing that no matter how hard we try, the "in-box" will never be empty. We can always find some task to do. Instead of stressing about it, we can enjoy the process.

This never-ending list of tasks makes setting priorities that much more important. Not infrequently, we procrastinate and delay the activities that are most important. The real stress is the dread of having some important task loom over us like a black storm cloud. Often, once we get started, we actually enjoy the task.

✎ Life Priority List

Take the time to list your life goals and priorities (such as education, family, health, and exercise). Then make a "to-do list," and then a daily schedule that includes the most important priorities. You can rank the items A (most important), then B, and finally C (least important). Make sure you include the A priorities in your day, every day. Do not think that marking things with an A ranking means they have to be hard work. Exercise, adequate sleep, and a relaxation exercise are examples of moderate, but advisable, A priorities.

In his book *Getting Things Done,* David Allen offers a strategy to deal with the "stuff" that comes across our desks. Simplified, he advises that as a given piece of material comes across your desk, quickly decide if it is or is not something "actionable." If it requires no action, decide whether it goes in the trash, or whether it should be kept in a reference file or in a "someday maybe" tickler file. If it is actionable and requires less than two minutes, do it at that time. In general, it is not worth spending extra time scheduling an action that takes only two minutes to accomplish. Just get it out of the way. (This strategy is useful at home as well as at work. Putting away a little piece of clutter as you notice it or replacing the used-up soap will help keep your house more efficient and less cluttered and will keep the other people in your house happier.) If you are not going to do a task right away, you can either schedule it for a particular time, put it on a to-do list, or delegate it.

It is important to include activities in your day that you enjoy doing. Psychologist Robert Ornstein and physician David Sobel talk about "healthy pleasures" as a way of keeping stress in check. These may include a variety of activities, from relaxing in a bathtub to taking a hike. Ideally, think of at least some activities that you enjoy that do not require a lot of time. Then include these activities throughout the day. More examples of healthy pleasures are listening to music, spending time with your pet, watching a sunset, getting a massage, giving a massage, making love, or just taking time out for a good hug, slowly enjoying a meal, reading a good book, viewing or creating art, gardening, and so on. Activities that include nature may be particularly helpful.

A recent study confirms that whether someone is a lottery winner or has relatively little money, happy people know to reward themselves with these simple pleasures. Less happy people rely on trying to buy items to make themselves happy.

✎ What I Like to Do

Take time now to list activities that you enjoy. Include some activities that do not take much time and can therefore be done even when you are busy.

1. _____
2. _____
3. _____
4. _____
5. _____
6. _____
7. _____
8. _____
9. _____
10. _____

Every minute you spend in planning saves 10 minutes in execution; this gives you a 1,000 percent Return on Energy!"

BRIAN TRACY

The use of a scheduling system will help prevent the stress of forgotten or delayed errands. Local office supply stores and bookstores usually sell items that vary from simple calendars to more elaborate scheduling systems. A relatively simple system is to have a calendar and a to-do list that you can update each day. A useful plan might be to draw a line through activities as they are accomplished and to circle the ones that are to be postponed until later. Some people use a PDA or palm-sized computer to manage their schedule.

> Jane had a staff of 50 people. She was constantly being interrupted with questions and felt she could not accomplish the project at hand. We discussed several strategies to deal with the problem. Many college professors schedule office hours for student questions. One possibility was to borrow this technique. For nonemergencies, people could contact her only during specific preset hours. Her secretary or voice mail would give people this information.
>
> We also discussed another strategy. If she were contacted with a problem she was too busy to handle, she would first empathize with the person's concern of urgency, then let him or her know that she understood the importance of the problem and wanted to give it the amount of attention that it deserved. I advised her to then schedule a time when she could give the problem sufficient attention. Frequently, in order to increase the efficiency of the meeting, she could give the person some preliminary instructions or "homework." For instance, the person might come up with an outline of the concerns, do preliminary research, or talk with another associate prior to the meeting.

Another method of increasing your effectiveness with time management is to learn to delegate responsibilities. Some people find letting go difficult, and even when they do delegate a task, they are sometimes too quick to reassume the responsibility. You may hear them say, "If I don't do it myself, it won't be done right."

Delegation can make your life a lot easier, if you train your helper or assistant properly. Allow people the time to learn the task and give them feedback when necessary.

⇨ *Delegation Practice*

Choose one task that you have always done yourself, either at work or at home, and delegate it to a coworker, a child, or someone else appropriate. Do not micromanage or revoke the task, but provide support as needed. Allow enough time to pass to see if the new person has handled the task or not. Were you surprised? Are there other tasks you can get off your plate?

Many people spend several hours a day watching television to "decompress." Go ahead and watch a television show that you like, but avoid spending hours "surfing" through the channels. Spending hours watching shows you don't enjoy—just to get up and realize all the chores are left to be done—does not relieve stress. Also, watching a lot of television violence does not contribute to long-term well-being. Be aware of what you feed your children's minds—and your own.

A study in the *Journal of the American Medical Association* examined the association of sedentary activity with obesity and diabetes in over 50,000 women. You might not be surprised to learn that each two-hour-a-day increment of sitting at work was associated with a 5 percent increase in obesity and 7 percent increase in diabetes. Interestingly, each two-hour increment of sitting in front of a television was associated with a 23 percent increase in obesity and a 14 percent increase in diabetes. Why was the television worse? It is unclear. It could be the commercials, encouraging you to eat, or a variety of other factors. Whatever the case, too much television is clearly not good for you.

Many families have a television in every room and habitually turn on the set as they walk into the room. Giving away a television or two may be an effective time management and stress management strategy.

⇨ Television Experiment

Strictly limit your television for one week. Stick to it, no matter how tempted you are to watch more. In order to make limiting TV time easier, you can try unplugging the television set or unhooking the cable line. If the television is small enough, you can try putting it away. By the end of the week, are you missing it a little less? How did you fill your newfound time? See if television seems less appealing the following week.

> Michael was a college student who came to an appointment complaining of back and abdominal pain. He had already been to several specialists and had multiple tests. He feared that the pains might be caused by some sort of cancer. I reviewed with him that the previous tests had eliminated the possibility of cancer. His pain was real, but the causes of it were irritable bowel syndrome and back spasm, both made worse by stress.
>
> We first explored Michael's thought processes. He would start thinking about how he was "overwhelmed" by his class assignments. I suggested that, when he noticed the thoughts that he was overwhelmed, he let those thoughts go. Instead of worrying about the entire semester of work, he now could focus on doing the next task. When he did this, he started actually enjoying the tasks that he had formerly dreaded. He also unplugged the television. If there was an occasional important show to watch, he plugged the television back in. However, with the set unplugged, there was less temptation to take an impulsive two-hour television

break from studying. Instead, after every hour or two of studying, Michael would spend 5 or 10 minutes stretching, listening to music, or playing with his dog. He also started to schedule regular times to swim and meditate. On Michael's next visit, his back pain was gone and he reported that his abdominal pain was "95 percent better."

The last time management tool is decreasing clutter. It can be quite stressful to spend 30 minutes searching for missing keys or a missing report. Organizing your environment at home and work can help decrease stress.

On being organized, a friend of mine tells this story:

It's something I learned when I had four young children and another six or eight coming to my home every day for child care. If I was organized, everything went well. But if I didn't make the effort—getting the school clothes together, cleaning the playroom, making lunches, and so on the evening before—the morning was inevitably full of stress, which would boomerang through the day. I am one of the most organized people I know as a result!

When friends and family were going through bad times, it would be inevitable that their houses were a mess, bills weren't being paid on time, kids had lost important papers, shoes, and so on. I would go over and start in one corner with them and just start cleaning, putting away, and organizing. Having things jumbled and disorganized just added to their problems. Knowing that the next day the kids would go off to school with both shoes and all their papers took away one very real stress!

One note of caution: If you are helping a friend or relative organize his or her home, be thoughtful in that organization. It is also important to communicate your plans. Otherwise you may add to your friend's stress instead of decreasing it. If your friend cannot find an important item when rushing to work, since it is in a drawer that only you know about . . . well, you get the picture.

Exercise

As we've discussed, stress has been described as the "fight-or-flight response," not the "couch potato response." Since your stressed-out body is screaming at you to act, blood and oxygen pounding through your muscles, it only makes sense that regular exercise is a good way to burn off some of that excess energy. Some people can use exercise only as needed; that is, the effects of a hard day at the office may be alleviated by a good jog after work. However, for health reasons and consistency, it is ideal to do exercise of some kind on most days.

You have two tasks in this section. The first one is to make exercise fun. If you are someone who is addicted to your lounge chair, "fun exercise" sounds like the ultimate oxymoron. But there is an exercise for everybody. If you get hives just thinking about jogging, find something else. Do you like walking, dancing, swimming, biking, hiking, racquetball, basketball, tennis? . . . come on now, I can't go on forever. Circle at least one or two of the choices.

✎ Fun Exercise List

Make a list of exercises that you might enjoy. Be creative as you brainstorm: Feel free to get specific. If you like dancing, what kind of dancing: aerobic dance class or jazz or ballroom? Do you like road bike, mountain bike, stationary bike, or all of the above? Do you like walking on your favorite hiking trail, walking on a treadmill as you watch television, or taking a brisk walk with a friend or spouse as you catch up on life? Do you like exercising while listening to funk on your MP3 player or while listening to birds singing? List your favorites, as well as ones you'd like to try.

1. _____
2. _____
3. _____
4. _____
5. _____
6. _____
7. _____
8. _____
9. _____
10. _____

Cool—one task done! The second task is to make exercise automatic. The type of exercise can vary, but the *choice* should be automatic. Find where exercise fits in your day. Does it seem impossible to fit exercise into your schedule? Don't give up easily. The ideal time might be first thing in the morning, at lunchtime, or after work. Try taking a regular walk with the dog or a baby stroller. If the weather is bad and you don't want to go outside, a home exercise machine might be helpful. Consider walking to the store or, if possible, biking to work instead of driving. When my twin boys were infants, either one or the other would often get cranky in the early evenings. Taking one of them out for a walk in a baby sling would calm the baby and give me a chance to get exercise. You might plan a similar exercise routine each day, or you might prefer variety. Either way, if you make exercise part of your daily routine, you are more likely to do it rather than just think about it.

✒ Schedule Your Exercise for the Week

Sunday:_____

Monday:_____

Tuesday:_____

Wednesday:_____

Thursday:_____

Friday:_____

Saturday:_____

With your exercise, you do not have to elevate your pulse excessively. Raising your pulse rate to 60–80 percent of your maximal predicted pulse for 20 to 30 minutes most days is sufficient. In order to calculate your maximal predicted pulse, subtract your age from 220. For instance, if you are 40 years old, your maximal predicted pulse would be 220 minus 40, which equals 180. Your target heart rate would 60–80 percent of 180, which equals 108–144. Your pulse can usually be felt at the thumb side of your wrist or at the groove on the side of your neck below the angle of your jaw (check only one side at a time). To calculate your heart rate, count the number of pulsations you feel in 15 seconds and multiply by 4. (See figures 5 and 6.)

Put another way, you don't have to run as hard as you can. Taking a brisk walk is excellent exercise. People over 35, or with medical problems such as heart disease, should discuss an exercise program with their health care provider before beginning.

Ted usually tried to go for a jog after work. However, he noticed that one thing or another always seemed to get in the way. One day, it might be additional paperwork from the job; another day, it might be a family obligation. Ted was in the habit of setting the alarm for 6:10 a.m. and hitting the snooze button once or twice

FIGURE 5
You can take your pulse by lightly placing the index and long fingers of one hand on the thumb side of the opposite wrist. Count the number of beats in 15 seconds and multiply by 4 to obtain the pulse rate.

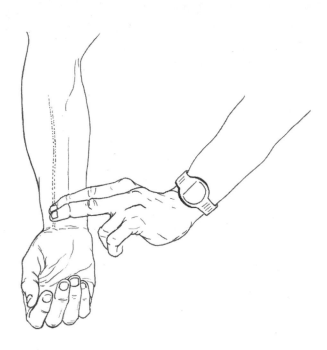

FIGURE 6
You may also take your pulse by lightly placing your index and middle fingers on the groove on the side of your neck (check only one side at a time).

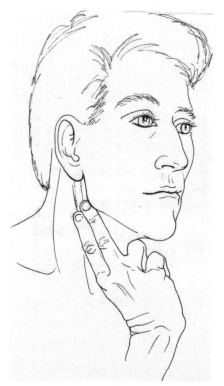

before getting out of bed. He would then go downstairs and make some coffee. He would slowly wake up and get ready to be at work at 8:00 a.m. One evening. he decided to try something different. He set his alarm 10 minutes earlier and visualized getting out of bed as soon as the alarm went off. The next morning he did just that. He put on his running clothes and was out the door in minutes, jogging in the crisp, fresh air. Ted felt so refreshed from his morning run that he found he did not need his usual coffee. In fact, the next week, he spent his morning "coffee break" relaxing with some fragrant herbal tea, instead of nursing his third cup of coffee. Once he began to experience the invigoration of exercise, he looked for new ways to add it into his life—not as a chore, but as a pleasurable activity. During the weekends, he soon began to take longer hikes and bicycle rides. He found that, as soon as he had recognized exercise as something that added genuine quality to his life, it was possible to fit it into his schedule.

Avoiding Excess Alcohol, Caffeine, or Drugs

Stan was about 30 years old and was suffering from what appeared to be severe panic attacks. Before prescribing the medications typically used for panic attacks, I asked him how much coffee he drank. "Three a day" was his answer. I told him that three cups of coffee per day could certainly increase a person's anxiety level. Then Stan clarified his response: It was three pots of coffee a day!

People have varying sensitivities to caffeine. Even a cup or two a day can cause problems for some people. Caffeine is also contained in many teas, chocolate, and some sodas. Although caffeine can precipitate headaches in some people, a sudden reduction in caffeine intake may also result in headaches or fatigue for a few days. Therefore, some people choose to gradually reduce their caffeine consumption, instead of suddenly discontinuing it.

Most of us have developed a somewhat warped sense of what a normal serving is. Does anyone really need to drink a 64-ounce soda with more than five times the caffeine and sugar of a standard 12-ounce soda? I used to wonder why a coffee shop would have sizes tall, grande, and vente. I thought, why not use the terms *small, medium,* and *large*? Then I heard someone order a short cup of coffee and discovered that a short cup of coffee is a conventional 8-ounce cup of coffee. In other words, even what most people consider the small size (tall) is 50 percent larger than a normal cup of coffee. I guess saying *tall, grande,* and *vente* sounds better than 1½ cups, 2 cups, and 2½ cups of coffee, respectively. Do not forget the humongous mugs people have at home and work. Is that two cups of coffee you thought you were drinking really five cups?

Keep in mind that different types of soda and coffee have different amounts of caffeine. Although you may find sources claiming that a cup of coffee has about 100 mg of caffeine, caffeine from certain shops may have 80 percent more per 8 ounce cup. Ounce per ounce, some caffeinated sodas have three times the caffeine of others. Thankfully, many of these comparisons can be done on Web sites such as www.wikipedia.org (look up "caffeine") and on the Web sites of the larger coffee-shop chains.

A glass or two of wine helps some people relax, but when alcohol is taken in excess, distress may worsen. Many heavy drinkers are surrounded by friends who also drink heavily, and they may have difficulty recognizing that they have a problem with alcohol. Recovery from alcohol addiction often requires that people find new social support groups. Alcoholics Anonymous is one group that serves this function well.

Several so-called recreational drugs can also cause increased
anxiety. Cocaine and amphetamines can cause severe anxiety and
panic. Even a single use of these drugs can cause a heart attack or
seizure. Illegal drugs are not the only drugs that make people anxious. Certain decongestants, asthma medications, antidepressants, and appetite suppressants can cause excessive anxiety in
susceptible individuals. If you suspect this type of problem with a
prescribed medication, discuss the issue with your doctor before
discontinuing it.

Nutrition

I went on a diet. Had to go on two diets at the same time 'cause
one wasn't giving me enough food.

BARRY MARTER

Good dietary habits are important for dealing effectively with
stressful situations. Low blood sugar can increase certain stress
hormones, which only makes sense: Hunger is one of the most ancient forms of stress. A nutritious breakfast is the best way to head
off the anxiety, irritation, stress, and shakes that accompany low
blood sugar.

Skipping breakfast is a big problem—and not just for your
stress level. Some people think that they'll lose weight by skipping
breakfast. Research by Mark Pereira (sponsored by the American
Heart Association) showed that people who regularly ate breakfast had a much lower incidence of obesity than people who did
not regularly eat breakfast. People who ate breakfast regularly
also had a lower risk of "insulin resistance." Insulin resistance, a
condition related to diabetes, is a risk factor for stroke and heart
attack. Eating a healthy breakfast low in saturated fats and sugars
further lowered the risk of obesity and insulin resistance. If there

is absolutely no time for a meal, a meal substitute (such as a protein drink or bar) is better than skipping breakfast completely.

Small, frequent meals keep your blood sugar steady, your stress down, and your energy up. It is best to eat more whole-grain foods and vegetables, and fewer refined carbohydrates. Refined carbohydrates include foods such as cake, sugar, white bread, white rice, white pasta, regular sodas, and fruit juice. (Eating fruit is much better than drinking the juice since there is more fiber in the whole fruit.) Refined carbohydrates have a high "glycemic index." That means a given amount of white rice or cake will increase your blood sugar more than the same amount of vegetables or whole-grain food. The higher blood sugar in turn leads to the release of more insulin from the pancreas, which in turn leads to a precipitous drop in blood sugar. And as noted earlier, a very low blood sugar may stimulate the release of certain stress hormones.

Mindfulness is an important tool for healthy and enjoyable meals. Too often, we eat, but barely taste the food. We might watch television, obsess over the workday, or compare the meal to an earlier one. Sometimes we may enjoy the first bite of food and then, instead of enjoying the rest, we spend the time planning to get more. As an alternative, we can learn from certain wine connoisseurs, who don't simply drink wine; they savor it—appreciating the color, bouquet, and every subtlety of the flavor. Bringing the same degree of mindfulness to other food and drink makes mealtime much more enjoyable. As you are eating and notice your attention has drifted, bring it back to the sensations of eating. When you have thoughts comparing the food or judging the food, let the thoughts go and just appreciate the intensity of the aroma, texture, and flavor in this moment. As you eat mindfully, you not only enjoy your food more, but you also tend to make healthier food choices.

Another modern-day problem is the limited time we sometimes give ourselves to eat. As our lunch hours get crammed with paperwork and errands, we tend to inhale our food. Make certain that you schedule adequate time to eat and enjoy your meals.

When you are trying to lose weight, it is important to be mindful of the decreasing sensation of hunger. Before eating, take some diaphragmatic breaths and notice if you have any sensation of hunger. If not, postpone eating, if possible. Often, we eat out of habit or to deal with stress, sadness, or other emotions. I also advise people interested in weight loss to stop eating every few bites, take some deep diaphragmatic breaths, and evaluate their level of hunger. Some people end their meal when they are "full," but by that, they mean "stuffed." The sign that you are full should not be that you can't possibly force another bite into your mouth! Rather, I advise people to stop eating as soon as the hunger sensation *begins* to subside. Put the food away or get up from the table to discourage mindless nibbling. The sensation of being full grows for up to 20 minutes after you stop eating. This style of eating encourages the healthy routine of eating small, frequent meals. Keep in mind that if you eat at twice the pace, but eat twice as much food, you have saved no time. You have only gained more indigestion, and more inches around your waist.

A guided eating meditation is included on Track 1 of CD 2.

Ethical Guidelines

It's hard to meditate when you've spent a whole day killing and stealing.

JACK KORNFIELD

It would indeed be hard not to be distressed if you've spent the day killing and stealing. We have all certainly acted in ways that we have regretted. However, committing yourself to behave according to some sort of reasonable ethical guidelines allows you to go about your day with less guilt and stress. All religions have rules of ethics, ranging from the Ten Commandments to the Buddhist Precepts and Eightfold Path. The simplest guideline may be the Golden Rule: "Treat others as you would like to be treated." However, it is also useful to have more specific guidelines, such as: no killing, no stealing, speaking wisely (avoiding lying, gossiping, slander, etc.), and avoiding sexual misconduct. Following ethical guidelines such as these should decrease our stress. In turn, as we develop our mindfulness and stress management, we will naturally want to act ethically.

Social Support

A friend divides your sorrows and multiplies your joy.

ANONYMOUS

There is nothing on this earth more to be prized than true friendship.

SAINT THOMAS AQUINAS

Our quality of life and ability to handle stress can be enhanced by a good social support system. The benefits of a good support system range from an increased resistance to colds to a longer life. Several studies have correlated an improvement in social support with a decrease in the incidence of heart disease.

It is more important to develop a few close friendships with people in whom we can confide than to have a long list of acquaintances. Our friends and our families are extremely important and should not be taken for granted. Be mindful to nurture your current relationships. Establishing new relationships can also be important. Participation in adult education classes, churches, synagogues, or any of a variety of other activities may help you meet people with common interests. If you enjoy hiking, join a hiking group to meet people with a similar interest. Varying your routine can give you the opportunity to meet new people. One patient of mine went to the same church every Sunday for many years. When he finally went to another church for a change of pace, he met the woman who became his wife.

Your Closest Friends

List your closest friends and family. Then, after each name, write an action that would nourish the friendship (spending regular time together, talking regularly on the phone, etc.).

1. _____
2. _____
3. _____
4. _____
5. _____

New Friends

List activities where you might establish new friendships:

1. _____
2. _____
3. _____
4. _____

When my wife was 20 weeks pregnant with our twins, she developed premature contractions. She starting having up to 12 contractions in an hour. We knew that, if delivery happened any time before 24 weeks, we would lose both of our twins, so her premature contractions were extremely stressful for us, to say the least.

We employed several strategies to help with this stress. Among the most important was relying on social support. We got support from her physicians. We did our research and strictly followed her doctors' recommendations. My wife was amazing. She followed the orders for bed rest very strictly and took medication to decrease the contractions, as prescribed. We asked for support from family and friends. We resisted the urge to be "polite" and not accept help. Friends cooked meals. Family visited and helped my wife with bed rest. We found a support group for pregnant women on bed rest and learned what we could from them. (The group is Sidelines, and information can be found at www.sidelines.org.) We prayed. My wife learned and did self-hypnosis, and she spent quiet time listening to relaxing music. When she relaxed in this way, she noticed that the contractions seemed to decrease.

We are extremely thankful that my wife gave birth to two wonderful boys. If you have had one new baby, you know how much work is involved. Of course, taking care of twins is even more work. If ever the lack of sleep and amount of work became difficult, the greatest tool that helped us manage the stress was our gratitude for having our two wonderful boys.

Our social support continued to be important after our boys were born. Our family and friends continued to offer help, and we continued to accept it. We joined the local Parents of Multiples group to help us with hints and support regarding raising twins.

People have a variety of emotions during a period of grieving, and these emotions frequently change. They may include shock, sadness, anger, denial, and/or guilt. Social support is important in coping with stress, and also in dealing with these other emotions. Even after time does some healing, an event or memory can suddenly change happiness to sadness. Sometimes, the oddest thing can stir a memory out of the blue, and the tears flow. As long as you do not resist the tears, the sadness eventually passes.

> When my father passed away, talking with family and friends was extremely helpful. My family and I took some time off work so we could just grieve together.
>
> Support from clergy was also helpful. During the funeral service, the clergyman said something that comforted me. My father could live on—not only in memories—if we made his great qualities our own. We talked of his kindness, honesty, and love of his family. If we made it a point to embody these qualities, our father would live on in us.
>
> During another religious service, I heard a question that, for some reason, comforted me. Someone asked: "If you could make the choice that no person currently living would ever die, but there could be no other baby born to enjoy life's pleasures, would you take that deal?" I would not take that deal. And somehow, that notion helped me be a little more accepting of the cycle of life and death.

Summary

You can manage your stress through a healthy lifestyle, which includes

- the creation of balance in your life;
- time management;

○ regular exercise;
○ proper nutrition;
○ the avoidance of certain drugs, and of excess alcohol and caffeine;
○ the maintenance of ethical guidelines;
○ the establishment of your friendships as a priority.

✎ List specific ways to improve your lifestyle.

10

Improve Your Communication

If you want to be listened to, you should put in time listening.
MARGE PIERCY

If there is any great success in life, it lies in the ability to put your-self in the other person's place and to see things from his point of view—as well as your own.

HENRY FORD

MUCH OF OUR stress centers on our relationships with others. Therefore, improving our ability to communicate should improve our ability to manage our stress. Carl Rogers, the father of "humanistic" or "client-centered" psychology, taught that there are three basic components of good communication: unconditional positive regard or acceptance, empathy, and genuineness. Unconditional positive regard or acceptance is illustrated by the following Rogers quote:

One of the most satisfying feelings I know—and also one of the most growth-promoting experiences for the other person—comes from my appreciating this individual in the same way that I appreciate a sunset. People are just as wonderful as sunsets if I can let them be. In fact, perhaps the reason we can truly appreciate a sunset is that we cannot control it. When I look at a sunset, as I did the other evening, I don't find myself saying, "Soften the orange a little on the right hand corner, and put a little purple along the base, and use a little more pink in the cloud color." I don't do that. I don't try to control a sunset. I watch it with awe as it unfolds. I like myself best when I can appreciate my staff member, my son, my daughter, my grandchildren, in this same way.

Unconditional positive regard has two elements. One is to be "mindful" as you listen to someone; that is, to be present and pay close attention to the other person during the conversation. The other involves the acceptance of a person as he or she is. People have different styles. Some are like a sunset: mellow and easy to be with. Others are like the Rocky Mountains: rough and gruff. The Rocky Mountains can be a beautiful and awe-inspiring place to visit. However, if you are in the mountains and spend all of your time wishing that you were watching a sunset at the beach, you will not be happy.

Accepting people as they are, and learning to enjoy their individuality, does not mean you accept everything they do. As a saying goes, you can "love the sinner without loving the sin." Accepting someone also does not require you to spend time with that person. If you are at a zoo, you may see a lion and really admire it, but don't jump into its cage. On occasion, one might hear of a woman whose husband repeatedly beats her, but she continues to stay with him because she says she loves him. In this case, it would be better to love from afar.*

---

*For brevity, I have oversimplified the predicament in which certain abused spouses find themselves. For further support, contact the National Domestic Violence Hot Line at 1-800-799-SAFE; for hearing-impaired TDD at 1-800-787-3224. For emergencies, dial 911.

Another key component to good communication is empathy. Empathy sometimes gets confused with pity, which is very different. With pity, you may look down on another person. With empathy, you put yourself in the other person's shoes. Empathy underlines our commonality. Even if we have not gone through a death in the family, we have all had losses and know what loss feels like. We may never know exactly what another goes through, but we can try to get close. In fact, one of the few good things about our painful times is that they allow us to identify more closely with another's pain. Sometimes, the best training a doctor receives is when he or she or his or her family member is a patient. Where there is an empathetic listener, both people in a conversation benefit.

Empathy is not only an effective communication tool but also an effective stress management tool in its own right. When we can try to see life from another's point of view, we may notice our own anger, hostility, and stress fading. Empathy allows us to be more patient with friends, family members, and strangers that we interact with throughout the day, as well as with people whom we've never talked to. I once had a discussion with a patient with severe emphysema who claimed he was so upset by slow drivers that he'd gone back to smoking. If this same patient had been able to empathize with the predicament of the other drivers, he might not have felt as compelled to jeopardize his own health.

In 1995, a man sped through an intersection in Baltimore after the light had turned red. He hit the driver's side of my mother's car and almost killed her. She fractured three ribs on each side, fractured her pelvis, and punctured both lungs. The injured lungs could not function correctly and predisposed her to subsequent life-threatening pneumonia. She spent two months in an intensive-care unit on a breathing machine—unable to talk—and an additional several months recovering. Miraculously, with the help of a dedicated medical team and a lot of prayer, she recovered. But as you might suspect, when she first resumed driving, she was nervous and sometimes drove slowly.

The next time you get annoyed at the driver in front of you, realize that he may have a good reason for his behavior. Empathy allows us to recognize that there are many other stories besides our own.*

Genuineness, the third essential component of good communication, follows naturally when unconditional positive regard and empathy are present. It is not genuine to tell someone how wonderful she is and to think simultaneously that she is a jerk. However, it is genuine to have a thought that someone is a jerk, let that thought go, and then relate to that person in an empathetic and accepting manner.

With empathy, acceptance, attentiveness, and genuineness, our ordinary conversations can be transformed into something warm, intimate, and beneficial to both parties. Even when the situation is sad, we can have healing conversations that bring us closer to one another.

In addition to the healing potential, there are other practical benefits of empathy. Let's pretend that your job is to make the schedules for two bosses: Boss A and Boss B. One day, Boss A tells you that you should schedule their appointments every 30 minutes. The next day, Boss B tells you that their appointments should be scheduled every hour; therefore, you schedule people every hour. Four days later, Boss A storms into your office and

---

*There is a very legitimate worry about drunk drivers and the high percentage of deadly accidents they cause. I have wondered if a lot of accidents and deaths are also caused by drivers trying to make it through the yellow light. Certainly, a lot of accidents are caused by sleep-deprived drivers. So, if you have been drinking, don't drive; if you are tired, pull over and rest; and if you see a yellow light, stop if possible. It's too easy to temporarily lose respect for the amount of damage, loss of life, and family pain that can be caused by the cars we drive.

yells, "What an idiot! Can't you do anything right? I gave simple instructions to schedule people every 30 minutes and you couldn't even follow them."

There are several ways to respond to this situation:

1. **You say** to yourself, "Poor me. I always get these unreason-able, awful bosses. I'll probably lose the job." (Let's call this the victim response—not very productive.)
2. **You say** to your boss, "You think I'm the idiot? You are the stupidest person I've ever met!" (The aggressive response—don't be surprised if you get fired and have trouble getting a good reference letter.)
3. **You say** to your boss, "Yes, Boss. No problem. I'll do it how-ever you want me to. Sorry to inconvenience you." At the same time you think to yourself, "Well, she wants people scheduled more frequently. Let's see how she likes having them scheduled every 10 minutes." (The passive-aggressive response—may be fun in the short term, but unproductive in the long term.)
4. **You say** to your boss, "I understand why you are upset. If I asked an employee to do something, and it looked as if he disregarded my request for no reason, I would be angry as well. However, shortly after you gave your instructions, Boss B told me to schedule people every hour. I assumed you were aware of this. If you and Boss B can decide to-gether on my instructions, I'll be happy to comply." (The empathetic response. Notice how you first empathize with your boss, so she feels acknowledged, and then ask her to empathize with you.)

Barbara was having a lot of trouble communicating with her nine-year-old daughter. Barbara felt the trouble was that they both had short tempers and would yell at each other. When I asked for more information, I found that Barbara complained that her daughter Robin would say things like "All the other mothers spend more time with their daughters." Barbara would argue that it was not true, since she knew that most of the mothers of Robin's friends had full-time jobs. Barbara needed to work full time to make ends meet. I suggested that the next time Robin said, "All the other mothers spend more time with their daughters," Barbara start her response by expressing empathy: "Robin, it sounds as if you are really frustrated that we don't spend more time together." And then she might go on to say, "I really would like it if we could spend more time together as well. However, I need to work to pay the bills. If you get most of your homework done at your after-school program, when I pick you up we could spend extra time together at the park."

Can empathy help with the stress of caring for infants and raising young children? When our twins were born, we tried to empathize with the newest members of our family. They did not cry to annoy us. If their crying was hard to deal with at 3:00 a.m. some morning, it was important to reframe the situation and to realize that the crying was our children's only way of communicating their needs. We learned to try one strategy after another—feeding? diaper change? sucking? burping? being held? being put down?—until we satisfied their need.

Toddlers are in the process of learning to deal with feelings of anger and frustration. One mother, Elizabeth, made the analogy of a toddler's feelings during a tantrum as being similar to the worst case of PMS that could be imagined. Additionally, a toddler has limited language skills to express his desires and frustrations.

In essence, it is like having PMS feelings, while most of your words come out garbled and incomprehensible. During tantrums, Elizabeth tries to keep that analogy in mind to help her empathize with her toddler. She then can better understand that her child needs help learning to deal with his intense feelings.

Here are some other guidelines for communication:

1. **Actively listen.** Be mindful when you listen and let go of distracting thoughts. Have you ever spoken to a person who looks past you as you speak and never really hears what you are saying? Perhaps you remember an argument when someone did not hear what you were saying. It's likely you found this type of conversation frustrating. When a learned rabbi was asked his definition of wisdom, he replied that a wise man knows how to learn from each person he meets. When you enter into a conversation with someone, learn what that person feels and thinks. Active, focused listening helps family, work, and social relationships. Both people in the conversation benefit from active listening. Even if a goal of the conversation is to present your viewpoint, it will be helpful to understand your communication partner's point of view first. Former U.S. secretary of state Dean Rusk said, "One of the best ways to persuade others is with your ears—by listening to them."

2. **You don't always have to be right.** Conversations are less productive when the only objective is to win. Go into a conversation with the objective of learning how the other person feels. Be open to learning information that may change your point of view.

We must love them both—those whose opinions we share and those whose opinions we reject. For both have labored in the search for truth, and both have helped us in the finding of it.

SAINT THOMAS AQUINAS

Instead of the goal of always being right, have as your goal communicating effectively. Take pride in your ability to communicate, not in your ability to insist on being right.

3. Instead of criticizing others, try expressing how you feel. You may try using "I" terms instead of "you" terms. When you say, "I feel . . ." and go on to describe your feelings, people listen and are less likely to get defensive. Also, no one can effectively argue against a statement about how you feel. On the other hand, statements like "You should not have acted that way" and "You were an idiot" are likely to elicit arguments and defensiveness. For example, compare the statement "You are inconsiderate" with the "I" statement "I was hurt when you insulted me in front of the group." The second statement is more likely to lead to productive communication, instead of a nonproductive argument. Consider the following examples:

○ How would you feel if someone were to say to you, "You were inconsiderate being so late"? Compare that with how you would feel if someone said, "When I didn't hear from you, I was afraid that you might have gotten into an accident. I care a lot about you, so please call the next time you are running late."

○ How would you feel if your spouse said, "I can't believe you are eating ice cream again. You know it's not on your diet"! Compare that with "I really care about you. I'm afraid that one day you'll have another heart attack and I might lose you. It really worries me when you eat a lot of high-fat foods."

○ How would you feel if someone said, "I feel that you are domineering." That statement might sound like a feeling, but it is really an opinion. Compare that with "I felt hurt when you did not give me time to express my opinion. I need a moment to let you know what I think about the issue." (In general, if you follow "I feel" with either *you* or *that*, you're not making the type of "I" statement I am recommending. For instance, "I feel that you are an idiot" is not considered an "I" statement! When you say "I feel that" instead of "I feel," you are expressing an opinion instead of a feeling.)

4. Both empathy and communicating empathy are essential components of effective communication. Before hearing advice or a lesson in someone else's philosophy, people usually want to be understood. Imagine that you have been struggling with a problem. If a friend just quickly volunteers a solution, you might think that he or she has not taken the time to fully understand the problem and is trivializing your stress. In general, it is best to communicate your understanding of the situation before volunteering advice. Feeling understood often makes someone feel better and more open to a suggestion, and often, feeling understood is all someone needs to feel better.

Sometimes, it is tricky to communicate your understanding. Just saying, "I know how you feel" may lead someone to respond, "How can you know how I feel?" One way to communicate empathy is to paraphrase. Effective paraphrasing does not mean parroting back what someone said. Rather, it means incorporating the key elements of both the content and the emotions of what that person said. After a friend tells you a dozen things that went wrong that day, you might express empathy by saying, "It sounds as if you had a frustrating day with one problem after another." In another circumstance, it might be much better to begin with "That is a stressful situation" before saying, "Just do _____ to fix the problem."

This strategy is important in talking with both adults and children. One might say to a young child, "That's silly to be upset about losing that stuffed animal; you have several others." The child is likely to become even more upset because you did not appreciate his or her feelings. Something might not seem important from an adult perspective, but it may seem extremely important from the child's perspective. You might do better if you said, "I know you really liked your giraffe. That was upsetting to you to lose it.*

Once in a while, people reach an impasse; neither person understands the other's point of view. Instead of fully listening while the other person is talking, each person spends that time planning how to "win" the conversation. Requiring paraphrasing in this type of conversation forces both parties to listen to each other and attempt to empathize.

⇨ **"Talking-Cup" Exercise**

The following exercise can be used to help two people move beyond an impasse in a conversation: Only one person is allowed to speak at a time. While this person is making a point, he holds an object such as a cup. The second person must accurately paraphrase the first person's point before she obtains possession of the cup and has a turn to make a point. Not infrequently, it may take a few attempts to accurately paraphrase a point. When the person making the point feels the point was accurately paraphrased, the cup changes hands.

5. It's not always about you. If you find yourself saying, "I don't deserve to be treated this way," you may indeed be correct. However, how you are treated is often not a consequence of what you do or do not deserve. Rather, it may largely be the consequence of what is going on with the other person. Instead of immediately becoming defensive, try being empathetic to the other's situation and challenges. Be open to learning what may be intentionally or

---

*For more information on talking with children, read *How to Talk So Kids Will Listen and Listen So Kids Will Talk* by Adele Faber and Elaine Mazlish. New York: Avon Books, 1980.

unintentionally contributing to the other's frustration or anger. What is he or she feeling? What does he or she need?

> Peter got home from work one Friday afternoon, after his wife Lisa had had a particularly difficult week. It is hard enough to take care of a sick child, but she had been taking care of two sick children that week, when she herself had also been very sick most of the week. Understandably, she was in a bad mood when Peter got home. Peter answered the phone, and it was a thoughtful friend of theirs. Peter described how his wife had "ripped his head off" as soon as he got home. Their friend said, "Go put your head back on and help out."

It is important not to take things too personally. It's better to be less defensive and more empathetic. Give people some slack and "go put your head back on."

6. Reframing allows you to listen to comments constructively, instead of defensively. It also helps you to find a positive meaning in what others say. One woman recounted an interaction with her loving, but sometimes critical, mother. The woman's fiancé had been a successful businessman, but his luck had changed. His business was bankrupt, and he had also declared personal bankruptcy. When the woman reluctantly revealed the news to her mother, her mother reacted by saying, "You have a knack for finding losers." This statement was very painful to the woman, until she reframed it in a positive light. She reasoned that her mother had meant to convey her disappointment since she wanted her daughter to find someone successful and to be happy. Once the woman was able to reframe her mother's initial comment and understand its motivation, she felt better. It is not uncommon for apparently negative comments to be motivated by caring and concern. Therefore, it often pays to look for the motivation behind a comment.

7. If you are not sure what the other person's point is, ask for clarification. Communication can be improved by asking for clarification not only of a specific statement, but also about the associated thoughts and feelings.

8. Listen to both the emotion and the words. When someone expresses his or her viewpoint in an emotional or loud manner, the tendency is to react by becoming argumentative. Instead of immediately getting argumentative or defensive, take a moment not only to listen to the words but also to consider the emotions implied and expressed. Remember that the intensity of the emotion is a loud signal that the issue is very important to the person with whom you are speaking. Therefore, take some extra time and patience to listen to what he or she is saying.

9. If at all possible, avoid saying something that could be interpreted as a threat. Most people (probably like yourself) tend to respond negatively to this form of communication. Just imagine your response if someone said, "Do this, or else."

10. Do not throw in the kitchen sink. That is, *keep to the topic of the current disagreement.*

11. Keep an internal locus of control. Do not blame others for your emotions. Your conversation will be more productive if you avoid blame in general. Using "I" statements can help you do this.

12. Sometimes writing issues down can help. Usually, it is best to address a concern as soon as you can. However, there are times when someone is not available to communicate when you are thinking about a particular issue or you need time to compile your thoughts. When you find yourself reviewing a conversation again and again in your head, list the main points of the conversation on paper. This activity allows you to quiet your mind more easily, since you may feel less need to rehearse the conversation continually in your mind.

To keep your marriage brimming
With love in the marriage cup,
Whenever you're wrong, admit it
Whenever you're right, shut up.

OGDEN NASH

It probably would not hurt to repeat this poem once a day. It's a humorous way of making the point that it is not wise to communicate with the sole goal of proving you are right. One of the most important messages in this chapter is to remind yourself to pause when you find yourself in this trap. Aim to fully understand the other person's viewpoint and communicate effectively. Do not take pride in always being right. Take pride in being a good listener and an effective communicator.

Denise had a difficult time getting along with her sister Alice. I asked for a specific example of one of their conversations:

DENISE: I was really hurt when you called me fat in front of other people.
ALICE: You always say things like that to me.
DENISE: I would never do that. You are so inconsiderate.

And then an argument and hard feelings ensued.

Suggestion of an alternative response for Denise: "I didn't realize that I've said things that have hurt you. If you see that I am doing something like that, let me know right away. I really will try my best not to offend you. I care about you, and hurting you is the last thing that I would want."

With this alternative response, Denise does not use "you" terms, and she does not insist on winning an argument.

Feedback

Everyone wants to be appreciated, so if you appreciate someone, don't keep it a secret.

MARY KAY ASH, Founder, Mary Kay Cosmetics

Feeling gratitude and not expressing it is like wrapping a present and not giving it.

WILLIAM ARTHUR WARD

It is helpful to learn to accept other people's behavior. However, sometimes it is useful to attempt to change another's behavior by giving effective feedback. Positive feedback is given to make it more likely someone will repeat a desired behavior. In contrast, negative feedback is given to make it less likely that someone will repeat an undesired behavior. Poorly delivered feedback can backfire by making people defensive, thus making a situation more stressful.

○ Feedback should not be insulting or demeaning. Demeaning feedback produces defensiveness and hostility instead of the desired results.
○ Feedback should refer to a person's behavior rather than a trait. For instance, instead of "You are clumsy," effective feedback might be "When you use the large drill, be sure to use both hands and use the left hand for the lever." Similarly, calling someone rude is usually less effective than asking him or her to let you finish a story before interrupting.
○ Feedback should be as specific as possible. Instead of saying, "You do careless work," you could explain which specific work project needed improvement and what specific improvements were needed. This precise information will be

much more useful in preventing a similar mistake in the future.

○ Feedback also needs to be understandable. Often, it is best to avoid jargon and technical terms.

○ Feedback should be well timed. In general, negative feedback should be given individually, whereas sometimes it is appropriate to give positive feedback in front of a group. Feedback should usually be given as soon after the event as possible. We may have assumed that we were doing a task well, and then long after the task was complete, we received some negative feedback. By that time, it was too late to make any changes, but not too late to be annoyed. Supervisors should give feedback frequently. There is an art, however, to determining how much is too much. There is an old expression: "Pick your fights." Continuous negative feedback or nitpicking can backfire by making people ignore all feedback, including the important stuff.

○ No one likes to hear feedback only when things go wrong. Does someone need to win the Nobel Prize before you say, "Good job"? A good hint for giving feedback, whether it be in raising children or talking to coworkers, is to catch someone doing something right. Don't wait for a heroic act! With young children, you might really need to be creative in that positive feedback: "You've been playing so well with your brother for the last 30 seconds." Positive feedback can be as effective as, or even more effective than, negative feedback. Positive feedback has an added bonus: The next time negative feedback is given, it is likely to be received more willingly and less defensively. No one who is working hard likes to hear only negative comments. All of the preceding points about feedback are applicable to positive as well as negative feedback. "You are conscientious" is a nice compliment, and compliments definitely have their place. However, telling someone the specific behavior you liked is more likely to increase the continuation of that behavior.

There is skill in receiving feedback as well as in giving it. Even poorly delivered feedback may contain a useful message. If someone offers feedback to you that is not specific or is about a trait rather than a behavior, you may be tempted to get defensive and perhaps even angry. Before reacting with anger, consider asking for clarification. Is there a specific behavior that should be improved? Also, do not listen only to the person's words. What is the feeling behind the communication? What is the need that the person may be expressing? By asking these questions and by asking for clarification when needed, you can avoid feeling insulted. You can also ascertain if the feedback contains useful advice.

Ann was getting frustrated with a coworker, Robin. At most of their group meetings, Robin would seem to nitpick Ann's performance. This was incredibly stressful for Ann. On my suggestion, Ann reframed the situation and realized that Robin, at times, actually had given some useful feedback. When Ann thought about it, she realized that what she really resented was that the feedback was given in a group setting. Instead of being angry at Robin, she thanked Robin for the feedback that was useful. She then requested that Robin give her feedback privately. Thereafter, Ann and Robin got along better, and Ann could actually use some of Robin's feedback, instead of just growing annoyed at her nitpicking.

Wendy was very frustrated about the performance of her employees. She complained that, when she would ask them to do a task, it would often be done incorrectly. I asked if she had checked with her employees to see why they were not getting the job done. She said that she had asked. However, what she had asked was "Did you not listen to me, or are you just not able to do the job?" I asked Wendy to consider checking into the problem in a way that would be less demeaning to her employees. I emphasized that it was more important to communicate effectively than to try to "be right." She had more success when she said, "It seems I am not effectively communicating what needs to be done. Is there a different or new way that I could discuss the assignment, so you understand it better?" Once she did give the instructions, she could check on whether her employee understood them. For instance, she could say, "I'm still not sure I am doing a good job getting my message across. This information might be confusing. To make sure I did get the message across, could you please tell me your understanding of what we discussed, before you get started on the project?"

Nonviolent Communication

Author and communication expert Marshall Rosenberg tells the story of taking a long pause before responding to one of his sons. He was struggling to find the words to communicate in a thoughtful, nonaggressive manner. His son, becoming impatient with the pause, said, "Daddy, it's taking you so long to talk." Rosenberg responded, "Let me tell you what I can say quickly: 'Do it my way or I'll kick your butt.'" His son said, "Take your time, Dad. Take your time."

Instead of reflexively acting, sometimes we need to take a second or two (or much longer) to come up with an effective way of communicating. It can be a struggle as we think about one insult or one "you" statement after another. Then, finally, we find the right words. Especially as we are first learning a new way to communicate, we may really need to pause to think about how we would like to respond. Old habits take some effort to break. However, if you want to improve your relationships at home and work, it is well worth the work.

Rosenberg espouses what he calls "nonviolent communication," or NVC. In short, NVC consists of four steps: (1) describing a problem in nonjudgmental terms; (2) describing the feelings involved (using "I" statements); (3) describing a need; and (4) making a specific request (not a demand).

⇨ *The Slow Response*

The next time you are about to respond during a stressful conversation, take the time to think about your answer. Try to follow the communication guidelines expressed in this chapter when you do respond.

In his workshops, Marshall Rosenberg has a unique way of illustrating two different styles of communication. He uses the jackal as a symbol of our usual nonproductive communication and the giraffe as a symbol of NVC (partly because the giraffe has the largest heart of any land animal). Then he can visually illustrate different ways of hearing by putting on different sets of fake ears. Putting on his jackal ears, he can show how a comment may cause an angry or sad reaction. When he puts on the giraffe ears, he not only listens to the words but also tries to find both the feelings and the needs that the other person is expressing. Suffice it to say, Rosenberg provides very important and entertaining workshops on communication. The image of actually putting on another set of ears drives home the point that there are different ways of hearing. When someone else makes a statement and you are just starting to get annoyed, can you put on a new set of ears? Can you listen not just to the words but to what feelings and needs are behind the words? To paraphrase Rosenberg, you can be criticized only if you are wearing the jackal ears, not if you are wearing the giraffe ears.

⇨ *Arrows into Flowers*

When the Buddha was about to obtain enlightenment, Mara shot 1,000 arrows at him. The arrows fell to his feet as flowers. Keep this image in mind the next time you think that someone is shooting verbal arrows at you.

Examining Intention

A man purposefully cuts another man with a knife. Is that a kind action or an unkind action? Jack Kornfield points out that, if the man is a robber intending to hurt his victim, it is certainly unkind to say the least. However, if the first man is a surgeon intending to help his patient, then the action is kind.

In any action, your intention is important. It is especially important in communication. As Kornfield points out, depending on the speaker's intention, "What do you mean?" has multiple meanings. If you are truly curious about what another means, you will communicate with a certain set of nonverbal cues (with both your gestures and your tone of voice). On the other hand, if you intend to be hostile and win an argument when you ask that question, you will have another set of nonverbal cues. This nonverbal communication is extremely effective in communicating your intention. In fact, one study at UCLA indicated that, in certain circumstances, up to 93 percent of communication effectiveness is determined by nonverbal cues.

When you pause to respond more thoughtfully, the first thing you might examine is your intention. Is your intention to communicate effectively and compassionately? Or is it to be right or to make another feel guilty? Whether you are aware of it or not, your intention is being communicated. Therefore, sometimes it is vital to pause, consider your intention, and "reset" it to communicate effectively and compassionately.

Even when we do not pause to check in on our intention prior to making a comment, we can reflect on it afterward. Once, my wife mentioned that our sons' educational toys had been left at their grandmother's house. My response was "That's the second time that's happened." In turn, my wife asked, "Why did you say that?" I reflected and realized that I was frustrated and had made the comment with the intention of making my wife feel bad. It was not a very skillful comment. She already knew about the error. My extra comment did not help. After realizing this, I apologized. When you notice that you have been communicating unskillfully, apologizing can stop the momentum that would otherwise lead to a destructive argument.

Are there ways to cultivate positive intentions? If we can, when the "moment of truth" arises and we are in the midst of a challenging conversation we are more likely to communicate compassionately. This topic will be discussed further at the end of the next chapter.

⇨ *Checking Intention*

The next time you are about to respond in a stressful discussion, ask yourself what your intention is. Before speaking, make sure that the intention is honorable and that the words match the intention.

The Art of Apology

Have you ever gone to apologize to someone and somehow you failed? You were trying to smooth things out, but before you knew it, an intense argument resulted. What is the explanation? Let's review a scenario:

You realize that you've acted inappropriately and go to apologize. Perhaps you feel bad. It is understandable and very natural to want to be understood and to want to describe why you acted the way you did. Here is the problem: Your attempt to be understood could easily be misunderstood as an attempt to justify your actions. "I'm sorry. I shouldn't have done ABC, but I did it because you did XYZ." And then the argument proceeds: "I did XYZ, because you did . . ." How can you apologize more skillfully?

First off, do you need to say anything to explain your motivations, or is it better to just apologize? Often, a simple apology without explanation works best. For instance, you might say, "I'm sorry. I won't do it again." Of course, if you promise not to repeat a behavior, you need to keep your promise.

In certain circumstances, you may feel it important to explain your actions. Perhaps you feel being better understood will help resolve the problem. Perhaps it will prevent future problems. If you feel the explanation is important, be mindful of the tendency for people to misinterpret your intention. Clearly state how you were wrong and apologize. Then you can clarify that you want to explain why you acted inappropriately. Remember to explain yourself with "I" statements. For instance, you might say, "I'm sorry. I really acted inappropriately. I am not justifying my actions, but I want to explain why I acted that way. It was a very long day at work. I was already frustrated and became more frustrated being reminded of the tasks I'd forgotten. I was way off base and apologize." Your apology does not need to be lengthy; just be aware of the pitfall of the "justifying apology."

Assertiveness

A "no" uttered from the deepest conviction is better and greater than a "yes" merely uttered to please, or what is worse, to avoid trouble.

MAHATMA GANDHI

Assertiveness is an important communication skill and a useful tool in dealing with stress. For our purposes, assertiveness means expressing your desires. It does not mean being aggressive, obnoxious, or rude. Many people manufacture stress for themselves by trying to please everyone, all the time. Saying yes to more tasks than you can comfortably handle, or saying yes to something you'd really prefer not to be involved in, is a sure recipe for stress. Assertiveness often takes the form of saying no when you don't want to do something. Even when you do not overextend yourself, the preoccupation with what others think may cause you much stress if you let it. It is important not to invest too much energy in worrying about what other people think of you. Let these excessive thoughts go, and do what you know to be right. As Shakespeare said, "To thine own self be true." Mahatma Gandhi said, "Happiness is when what you think, what you say, and what you do are in harmony." It is more important to follow your own sense of integrity and morality than to win others' approval.

Henry was performing well at work, but he found himself increasingly busy and stressed. As soon as he finished one project, he was assigned two more. Before he knew it, he was working 70 to 80 hours a week, and other areas of his life were suffering. He came to me complaining of palpitations and anxiety. Henry finally realized that it was rare to find a boss who would start a conversation by saying, "Take it easy; you've worked too hard already." When Henry voiced his desires in a polite, yet assertive, way, his boss was more than willing to accommodate Henry's request for a decreased workload. The palpitations decreased, and Henry had the chance to develop other parts of his life—including a new relationship.

Let's look at the above example more closely. Henry had several options:

1. Give in and accept any added work his boss would give him (passive response).
2. Angrily call his boss inconsiderate (aggressive response).
3. Politely, yet firmly, advise his boss that his plate was already full with other tasks (assertive response). Notice how each of the following assertive responses might be appropriate, so Henry could have some time off work:
   - "I'm already busy with two other projects, so I don't think that I'll have time for the new project."
   - "I'm doing the Smith and Jones project now, and I need to be home by 6 p.m. tonight. If you would like me to work on the new project, I'll have to postpone the others. Which project would you prefer that I complete today?"

We cannot count on a boss, coworker, or spouse to automatically try to decrease our stress load. It is essential to realize that, if we don't speak up for ourselves, often no one will.

The Clerk Is Not a Jerk

I remember, many years ago, reading a book that espoused the saying "The clerk is a jerk." What the author meant was that if you want to get something of value from a store, like a refund, you should seek the manager and not just settle for a negative response from a store salesperson or clerk. It may be true that, if you do not get satisfaction from a salesperson, talking with the manager will be helpful. However, far too often people do not treat staff members at a place of business with respect. As the saying goes, "You catch a lot more flies with honey than with vinegar."

When you deal with people with respect and a caring attitude, you will accomplish much more, and both of the parties involved will be less frustrated. You can always ask to speak to a supervisor later, but you may be surprised by what can be accomplished by being pleasant and nonthreatening to other employees first.

Keep this in mind, too, when talking to people on the phone. It is often too easy to forget that there is another real person on the other end of the line.

Extra Bonus of Skillful Communication

The communication hints will help you before you utter your first word. Consider the example of a fictional John and Mary who need to accomplish Tasks A, B, C, D, and E. John doesn't do his share of the work. Mary fumes, thinking, "John is so selfish and inconsiderate." She gets angrier and angrier as she thinks about this and plans to discuss her concerns with John. She then realizes that calling John selfish and inconsiderate may not be the most productive start to a conversation. Therefore, she thinks about how to communicate skillfully. Mary plans to say, "John, I feel really frustrated. So far, I have done Tasks A and B on my own. Would you please do Tasks C and D? Then we can do Task E together." Even before she says her first word to John, the communication hints have helped Mary become less angry and frustrated. Effective communication is not the only way to deal with anger and frustration. The next chapter will teach a variety of other effective skills.

Summary

Throughout this chapter, we have discussed a variety of communication skills. By effectively implementing these skills, you will improve your relationships with people in all aspects of your life. If you practice acceptance, empathy, genuineness, and assertiveness, your life will become less stressful and more fulfilled.

✐List ways you can improve your communication at work and home.

11

Deal with Anger and Frustration

Holding onto anger is like holding on to a hot coal with the intent of throwing it at someone else; you are the one that gets burned.

BUDDHA

If we could read the secret history of our enemies, we should find in each man's life sorrow and suffering enough to disarm all hostility.

HENRY WADSWORTH LONGFELLOW

ANGER, HOSTILITY, IRRITATION, impatience, and frustration are emotions that certainly increase our level of distress. When these emotions run amok, the result is disastrous! Increased risk of heart disease, ruined relationships, and even violence follow.

The country of Tibet was invaded by China in 1949. By some estimates, 6,000 Tibetan temples were destroyed and a million Tibetans died as a result of the Chinese occupation. The Dalai Lama is the spiritual leader of the Tibetan Buddhists. "When asked about his apparent lack of anger toward the Chinese . . . the Dalai Lama replied something to the effect that: 'They have taken everything from us; should I let them take my mind as well?'" The

Dalai Lama realized that if he were to harbor anger and resentment against the Chinese, he, not the Chinese, would be giving up peace of mind. The Dalai Lama continues to work toward his goal of a free Tibet, but without anger dominating his mind.

How do we deal with our anger? One of the most effective methods is mindfulness. Fighting the anger and wishing it away can just make us angry about being angry. As discussed in depth in Chapters 4 and 5, when we welcome our present-moment emotions, thoughts, and sensations, the next moment brings a new experience.

Another important skill in dealing with anger is empathy. If you are angry at someone, try your best to put yourself in that person's shoes. You may not imagine acting the way another person has acted, but you may be able to understand his or her motivation. You may be able to empathize with the frustration, anger, despair, or misunderstanding that leads another to act in a certain manner.

The next time you start fuming about the guy who cut you off on the freeway, remember a time when you mistakenly took another's right of way. When you get annoyed by someone, do your best to try to imagine what it would be like to be in her or his position. It's important to remember that when people are rude, they are usually suffering in one way or another.

When I'm on the freeway, I usually let people change lanes or get onto the freeway in front of me. I would sometimes get a little annoyed if others did not treat me with the same courtesy. One day, in a Washington, D.C., rush hour, I was following my brother-in-law. I was not familiar with the area. So as not to get lost, I tried to stay close behind his car and tried not to let other cars get between us. It occurred to me that when a driver would not let me into traffic, there might be a similar reason. The next time I was not let into traffic, I empathized that the other driver might be following his friend in a strange city.

🖎 Dealing with Frustration and Anger through Empathy

First, think of a situation in which you were angry at or frustrated by a person you know. How could you have empathized with that person's situation?

Next, think of a frustrating situation in which you do not know the other person involved (such as another driver on the road or a cashier). Although you do not know much about that person's life, imagine circumstances in which you could empathize with how that person has acted.

The weak can never forgive. Forgiveness is the attribute of the strong.

MAHATMA GANDHI

Another way to deal with anger is through forgiveness. Our families and friends are too important for us to continue harboring resentment. If you hold a grudge, your psychological well-being is negatively affected. We have all acted inappropriately at one time or another. We also have had people treat us inappropriately. They may have said or done something that was really off base. Being able to forgive is one of the most important qualities we can have in our relationships and for our own health.

A useful analogy to keep in mind is anger being like a storm. Even when people care about each other, once in a while they lose their tempers. The anger can blow into their lives with the ferocity of a rainstorm. However, when the storm of anger is over, it is over.

I clearly remember times in my life when I was angry and said something I should not have—something I did not mean that upset another. I can also think of misunderstandings when someone else said something I found very rude and offensive. My initial inclination was not to let bygones be bygones. It was to hold a grudge—a really good grudge. I recall when I was annoyed enough by someone's outburst that my annoyance really had the potential to ruin a whole family vacation. In that kind of situation, it pays to remember the analogy of an argument to a storm. In anger, we may act inconsiderately or make statements we do not mean, but then the storm is over. Forgiveness and "making up" may be even more beautiful than a rainbow after a storm. Our families, our friends, our coworkers, and the rest of the world could use a good, healthy dose of forgiveness.

For good reason, forgiveness is discussed in most major religions. Its importance is discussed in Christianity, Islam, and Hinduism. In Judaism, there is a Day of Atonement on which one fasts and asks for and gives forgiveness. There is also a Buddhist forgiveness meditation.

Forgiveness Meditation

In this meditation, we recognize that all people, knowingly and unknowingly, have harmed themselves and others. Get comfortable and close your eyes. Spend a few moments focused on your breath. Then, say to yourself, "May I be forgiven for any harm I have caused others either knowingly or unknowingly." Then, go on to say to yourself, "May I be forgiven for any harm I have caused myself either knowingly or unknowingly." Finally, say, "I forgive others for any harm they have committed against me, knowingly or unknowingly." When repeating these phrases, you may notice a decrease in your tendency to get stuck in feelings of anger, as well as a corresponding decrease in your stress.

There are other meditative approaches to dealing with anger. Sometimes, we obsess about an incident until we get angrier and angrier. Every time we tell the story and blame someone else, it is as if we are pouring oil on the flames of our anger. If left to its own devices, anger behaves more like a bouncing tennis ball. Anger over an event may return repeatedly, but each time it comes up, the intensity of the anger decreases, just as the tennis ball bounces lower each time. Finally, the energy is dissipated. When you stop blaming others for your emotions and just notice the physical sensations and thoughts associated with anger, the anger will more quickly dissipate. If you feel a knot in your stomach, it might be helpful to meditate using the mantra "Breathing in, I notice tightness in my abdomen . . . breathing out, I ease the tension in my abdomen." (Note: This technique is for temporary mild discomfort associated with anger. For severe or persistent physical discomfort, or for any chest discomfort, please consult your physician.) If you are too upset to sit still, consider a walking meditation. At times, even more vigorous exertion or exercise may help.

It is important not to just sit there and let your anger stew to a point where it eventually explodes. The above guidelines will help you deal with anger.

Additionally, it is helpful to address the circumstances surrounding the anger. In other words, communicate your feelings and address the situation before you get extremely upset. Be mindful of the assertiveness and feedback skills discussed earlier. If, for some reason, you cannot communicate about the problem right away, writing the issues down can help to decrease the likelihood that you will repeat the thoughts again and again, since you know the points are already on paper. Also, you will have the opportunity to think about how you want to communicate effectively, instead of just re-acting in a way that could inflame the situation.

Another way to deal with anger is to reframe a situation. As dis-cussed in Chapter 6, when you encounter someone who is rude, instead of dwelling on how terrible he is, think about how that person may be suffering in one way or another.

On one episode of the television show *Survivor,* toward the end of the game, one of the contestants voiced her feelings about an-other contestant, telling her that if she were dying of thirst in the desert, the first contestant would rather see her die and be eaten by vultures than give her a drop of water. *This was about a game!* How often do we overreact? I have seen people unleash a torrent of anger about a relatively small matter. Does the person you are angry with deserve such hostility? Is that person so evil?

In *The Art of Happiness,* the Dalai Lama describes other ways of dealing with anger. When people first fall in love, they tend to see only the positive traits in the other person. In a similar way, when we become angry with someone, we fixate on that person's negative traits. By deliberately listing that person's positive traits, we can decrease our anger. Your boss may be very stern, but what good qualities does she possess?

✐ Positive Quality Exercise

Next time you are angry with someone, list two to five good qual-ities about that person:

1. _____
2. _____
3. _____
4. _____
5. _____

Now note if your feelings have changed at all.

The Dalai Lama also stresses the importance of learning patience. He reminds us that people who frustrate us, or even wish us ill, are also the ones who give us the opportunity to learn the vital skill of patience.

Yet another way to deal with anger is to channel your feelings productively. That is, use the feelings to benefit your own or another's well-being. If you smoke, for example, you could use your anger over the hold cigarettes have on you to give you the strength to quit smoking.

Few experiences in life are more emotionally difficult than a parent's dealing with the death of a child. How can anyone deal with such anger and grief? In several instances, parents have done something productive with that anger. For instance, many children have died because their car safety seats were improperly secured. The parents of one of these children helped to publicize the prevalence and seriousness of this problem. By doing so, they saved many young lives. By using anger productively and nonviolently, we can create changes like this one and also work against a variety of societal injustices, as was done in the 1960s civil rights movement.

I feel incredibly blessed to have my two wonderful sons. They have given me immeasurable joy. Supervising twins, however, certainly has its frustrating moments as well.

For instance, I can remember putting sunscreen on them when they were two. This might not seem like a very difficult task, but when it involves two-year-olds who either do not want sunscreen or want to do the whole application on their own, the task can become a major challenge.

During one such episode with the boys, I noticed my frustration starting to increase. I thought about the typical process of making anger worse and holding onto it. We might feel physical sensations like tightness in our abdomen or jaw. These sensations are typically followed by thoughts like "I am angry," or "I am really frustrated." Since anger and frustration are often considered negative emotions, we often justify the emotions to ourselves. We tell ourselves the story that we feel both created and justified the anger. Each time we tell the story, we get more and more angry (or more and more frustrated). Instead, by just accepting our feelings, and not being compelled to repeatedly justify them, we give the anger or frustration the opportunity to quickly dissipate.

Before my frustration had a chance to build, I took some diaphragmatic breaths and chuckled. I realized that my twins were two wonderful teachers. By learning to patiently watch two active young boys, I would learn skills that I could use in many other areas of my life.

Since then, before I get too frustrated, I catch myself and think of my two wonderful little teachers, enjoy a nice breath, and laugh. Of course, when I once said something out loud about my two little teachers, they said, "Dad, we are not little teachers; we are big boys!"

When I find myself frustrated in other situations, thinking of people as my teachers can bring a smile to my face and a little creativity in trying to deal with the situation.

Language and Anger

"That which we call a rose, by any other name would smell as sweet;" or so said Juliet. However, if Romeo had had a different last name, the story of *Romeo and Juliet* might have turned out quite differently! Our words and language are extremely important. Even in our thoughts, the words we choose can make a big difference in how we feel.

In Chapter 6, we discussed the importance of an internal locus of control. We explained that saying, "You made me sad'" or "I am sad because you are late" implies an external locus of control. That language gives you only one choice of how to feel. If you want to have a more internal locus of control, you might say, "You were late and I was sad." There is another type of phrase unique to anger. We don't say, "I'm sad at him" or "I'm happy at her." If we did, people would look at us as if we were from Neptune. However, we do say, "I'm angry at him!" What's the implication of those words? He caused the anger! We were just standing around, minding our own business and he forced us to be angry. We had no choice in the matter.

How can we deal with our anger if we blame someone else for it? So, instead of "I'm angry at him," we might just say, "I'm angry."

In fact, we can do even better than "I'm angry." By using the common language convention of "I am angry," we imply that the emotion defines us. Instead of I am Jay Winner, I am angry! Obviously, there is more to us than our current emotion, but one wouldn't surmise that from the phrases "I am angry" or "I am sad." More accurate might be "I notice anger" or "There is sadness." Then we can notice the emotion with curiosity and interest. This approach applies to all emotions, but it is especially important with anger. Let's be practical: In day-to-day life, it is impossible never to say or think phrases like "I am angry." Just be aware of what you are saying and thinking, and when it is appropriate, rephrase your language.

⇨ Modify Your Language

Next time you think either "I'm angry because he ____" or "He made me angry" or "I'm angry at him," try restating the phrase: "He did ___ and I notice anger." (You can use the same type of phrasing to describe another emotion such as sadness.) Mindfully notice the anger and any associated physical sensations and thoughts. Then mindfully pay attention to a few breaths. Do you notice any difference in how you feel? Is there any change in the intensity of the anger?

Cultivating Compassion

Think about a time when you were feeling very loving and compassionate. I'm not talking about possessive, jealous, or romantic love. I'm referring to the wonderful feeling a parent might have for a child or a pet owner might have for a pet—the feeling that makes you want to do anything for your loved one. Of course, there are the times when your child puts an ice cream sandwich in the VCR or the dog mistakes your best shoes for his chew toy. Those times aren't warm and fuzzy, to say the least. But think of the feeling you have when your child says out of the blue, "I love you," or your dog nuzzles you at just the right time, or your friend says just the right thing to comfort you and gives you a hug. These are the times when you feel as if you would do anything to help someone, not because you should or it's the right thing to do, but just because you naturally want to do it.

❖ *Remembering Love*

Before reading any further, think of a time like that. Close your eyes and picture the scene as vividly as possible. Remember what you felt like when you experienced those feelings of loving-kindness and compassion. It felt really wonderful, right? When you felt loving, you weren't feeling stressed-out or angry. In fact, just remembering times like these makes us feel good.

As a general rule, when you experience loving-kindness, compassion, empathetic joy, and equanimity, you don't feel stressed out, angry, and frustrated. So if you don't want to be stressed-out and angry, learn how to cultivate loving-kindness and compassion. One piece of good news is that the practice of mindfulness that you have already learned will, in itself, increase loving-kindness and compassion. There are, however, other types of meditation (derived from the Buddhist tradition) specifically designed to cultivate these states.

In 2004, Richard Davidson studied Buddhist monks who were proficient in this type of meditation. The latest equipment, both functional MRI scans and EEGs, was used to study the monks. Results? The measurements were unlike those ever recorded: The monks were off the scale in the areas of happiness and compassion! The monks had changed the way their brains functioned.

By regularly practicing the meditations below, you will actually change your brain to increase happiness and compassion, and to decrease stress. (As you learn these meditations, it's worth pondering what the world might be like if more people became adept at these practices.) We spend a lot of time learning a variety of skills, hoping they will bring happiness. Why not spend time practicing skills that are scientifically shown to actually increase your happiness set point? Let's briefly discuss meditations on loving-kindness, compassion, and empathetic joy. Since the loving-kindness meditation is so useful, I have included two versions: a guided one on the CD and another nonguided version.

⊙ *Loving-Kindness Meditation. Disk 2, Track 4.*
Length: 14¹/₂ minutes.

Find a quiet spot where you won't be disturbed. Play the CD track and follow the guided visualizations.

❖ *Loving-Kindness Meditation*

Sit or lie down in a comfortable position. Close your eyes and visualize an image that brings forth loving-kindness. It could be an image of one who has been loving toward you, or it could be the image of holding a newborn baby in your arms. Imagine the scene as vividly as possible.

Next, visualize a person whom you naturally feel affection toward and say to yourself words such as "May you be safe and protected. May you be happy. May you be healthy. May you live with ease." (Living with ease means not removing all the challenges in life, but living joyfully without the sense of struggling.) Say the words at your own pace, and try to say them with meaning. You can modify the wording so that it is most meaningful to you. After you say each phrase, feel the physical and emotional effect of just having said it. If you would like, you can imagine hugging the person or holding his or her hand. Next, say similar phrases to yourself: "May I be safe and protected. May I be happy. May I be healthy. May I live with ease." If it is difficult to direct these phrases to yourself, you can imagine yourself as a small child and say those phrases to that child. Again, after each phrase, feel the effect of the phrase. Then, say the phrases while visualizing someone you might feel more neutral toward; perhaps someone you don't know well. Then say the phrases to someone you may have had some negative feelings toward. It is probably best not to pick out initially the person for whom you have the most negative feelings. You might start with a person whom you have found mildly irritating. Another option is to visualize that person with you and say words such as "May we be safe and protected. May we be happy," and so on.

Keep in mind that by wishing someone well, you are not necessarily approving that person's behavior. You are acknowledging that all of us really just want to be happy. Sometimes, we have been skillful in our attempt—bringing happiness to ourselves and others. Other times, we have been misguided and unskillful—bringing ourselves and others suffering. By keeping in mind our common wish, to just be happy, and our challenges, we can still offer the above wishes.

Traditionally, in a loving-kindness meditation (also known as a Metta meditation), one then offers the same phrases to a whole community and then to all beings. You might take 20 minutes or so to run through the whole sequence as described above. To make it easier to visualize people, you can keep their pictures by you as you do this meditation. However, you can also do a "Mini-Metta meditation." Prior to going into an appointment with someone, you might pay mindful attention to a couple of breaths and then say those phrases to yourself about the person you are about to meet. The 10 or 20 seconds it takes may help your meeting go more smoothly. You can even practice a little Metta as you walk down the street.

❖ Compassion Meditation

To cultivate compassion toward someone who is suffering, do a similar meditation, but imagine the one you know and say phrases such as "May you be free from suffering and the cause of suffering." Similar phrases can be said to yourself and to all beings.

At times, we are distressed by jealousy. Someone else gets the raise that you thought you deserved, and you steam. Someone else grabs the parking place that you had your eyes on, and the snake of jealousy bites. A meditation on empathetic joy can be thought of as antivenom for the snakebite of jealousy.

Young children are quite commonly jealous when another gets something. When this was once happening with my twins, I said to them, "Mommy and Daddy get to be twice as happy as you boys. Would you like to be twice as happy?" That question got their interest. I continued, "When something good happens to me, I get happy. However, I also get happy when something good happens to you. So I can be happy twice as often. You are already happy when something good happens to you. If you want to be twice as happy, you can also be happy when something good happens to your brother. You can practice this by saying to him, with meaning, 'I am happy for you.'"

❖ Meditation on Empathetic Joy

When something good happens to someone else and you feel jealousy begin to raise its head, say the following phrase, and direct it toward the object of your jealousy: "I am happy for you. May your good fortune and happiness continue. May it grow. May it increase." If you like, you can try first saying the phrases to one with whom you have a natural affinity (like a child).

If we look closely at our jealousy, we can see how silly it is. People become jealous of others' fame or fortune. When we get to know someone well, we see that those things do not bring happiness. The skills that nurture happiness are the very skills you have been learning to deal with stress. Through mindfulness, empathy, forgiveness, and cultivating compassion, we learn to deal with our anger.

🖊List ways to deal with your anger and frustration.

12

Take the Stress
out of Decisions

When you come to a fork in the road, take it.

YOGI BERRA

FOR SOME OF us, the times of greatest stress involve making decisions. We need to make many decisions throughout the day—some big, some small. It seems that, as our society becomes more advanced, the number of decisions we must make increases. The decisions range from what kind of toothpaste to buy to where we are going to live or work. We can keep in mind several ideas to help ease some of the stress involved in decision making.

⇨ Depressurizing Decision Making

The next time you are faced with an important decision, try to depressurize the situation by applying as many of the following as are appropriate:

1. **Most decisions** are not permanent. If you try something out and you don't like it, you can often change your mind. It may be inconvenient to change your mind and, in some

cases, not possible. Keep in mind, however, that many decisions are not final.

2. **Ask yourself,** "Will this decision matter in 10 years?" The answer, often, is no. This question will put the many decisions in perspective.

3. **If a** decision is hard to make, usually both choices compare closely in their virtues, so you can't go too wrong either way. If one choice were much better than the other, the decision would be easy!

4. **Remember the** concept of internal locus of control. Our happiness and peace of mind will be most influenced by internal factors such as our attitudes and our willingness to focus on the present. We probably can be happy or sad whether we live in Kansas or California, or whether we go to one college or another. We can frequently view our decisions as two alternatives that we could be happy with, as opposed to thinking that all of our happiness depends on the right decision.

Decision-Making Strategies

Half the worry in the world is caused by people trying to make decisions before they have sufficient knowledge on which to base a decision.

DEAN HAWKES

Once you've decreased your anxiety over the decision, you can employ the following decision-making skills to further decrease your stress—and hopefully to help you make a better choice.

1. **As the** Dean Hawkes quote implies, doing the necessary research is important. For instance, a book or the Internet may have information that could help with your decision. Be

creative in where to look for advice. Ultimately, the decision may be yours, but seeking the advice of others or discussing the options with others can be helpful. Seek someone who is an expert in the field or someone who has had to make a similar decision. You can also discuss the decision with other people who will be affected by its outcome. Some of the people to consider consulting include your family, your friends, your coworkers, a counselor, a member of the clergy, or a doctor. President Woodrow Wilson said, "I not only use all the brains that I have but all that I can borrow."

2. **Make a** list of pros and cons. Sometimes, decision making is easier when the advantages and disadvantages of each course of action are on paper. Writing the issues on paper will also decrease the tendency to argue the points over and over in your head.

3. **At times,** the best course of action is sitting with or sleeping on a decision, rather than worrying. Have you ever struggled with a decision, and then suddenly, something happens or an idea occurs to you, and the best choice becomes clear? This is a common phenomenon. If a decision needs to be made now, don't procrastinate. However, time is frequently available to consider the options. Instead of spending this time worrying, acknowledge that certain choices may become clearer on their own with a little time. Give yourself the permission to sleep on or sit with the decision. (Of course, in the meantime, you will do the necessary research, make your list of pros and cons, etc.).

4. **In times** of extreme emotional turmoil, it may be best, if possible, to postpone important decisions. For instance, when faced with the recent loss of a loved one, you may find it difficult to rationally weigh the pros and cons of a complicated decision.

5. **Brainstorming on** your own or with another person can be helpful. If you have two obvious choices, brainstorming will likely produce additional ideas. The first step is to come up with as many options as you can, no matter how impractical they might seem. You may ask a friend or group of friends, coworkers, or an organization to help. Afterward, you can critically analyze each choice to come up with a smaller, more practical list that may include more than your initial two options.

6. **Focusing on** the values involved in the decision and then weighing those values can be helpful. For instance, some decisions may involve the choice between a job with a higher salary and another that pays less but would be more fulfilling in other ways. Considering the 40 or more hours per week you may be at your job, a more fulfilling one may be more important. However, if earning less means more difficulty actually putting food on the table, the additional fulfillment might not be as important.

7. **The importance** of integrity cannot be overemphasized. Don't waste your time feeling guilty. To quote Abraham Lincoln, "When I do good, I feel good. When I do bad, I feel bad. That's my religion." Make the decision you can be proud of, and feel good about it. With certain decisions, you simply know what is right. Do it. Think about what your guiding principles are. For example, "Do not do any harm, and if possible, try to help others." If you are religious, consider what you think God would want you to do. Alternatively, you might ask yourself, "What course of action would I be proud to discuss with my children?"

8. **Pretend you** have made one of the choices, and ask yourself, "How do I feel?" Now pretend you have made the other

choice and ask the same question. This may be one way to access your "gut feeling" or intuition.

9. **Sometimes, a** decision is more difficult when there is a lot of static in our minds. If your mind seems to be racing, meditate, take a walk, or practice a walking meditation. These activities can help clear your mind and enable you to make a better decision.

10. *Fred had another strategy for dealing with business decisions. Sometimes, two people would offer him a deal and he could accept only one of the offers. He found that letting both parties know when the decision was close often helped him make the decision. One of the parties would frequently go that extra mile for the business deal.*

13

Improve Your Sleep

People who say they sleep like a baby usually don't have one.
LEO J. BURKE

STRESS AND SLEEP have an interesting relationship. A good night's sleep is very beneficial for handling stress. However, when people are very stressed, they often have trouble sleeping, which causes a negative feedback loop. How much sleep do you need? The simple answer is that you need enough sleep to feel rested. For some people, that can mean 5 hours; for others, 10. An average is around 8 hours. In general, people tend to need less sleep as they age.

In 1991, one research study compared several insomnia treatments for people over 65. One group received one of the most popularly prescribed sleeping pills of the time (temazepam; brand name, Restoril). A second group was given recommendations for changing their behavior at bedtime, while a third group received both the behavioral recommendations and the medication, and the final group received only a placebo. The only groups with long-term benefit were the groups that were given the behavioral treatments. In 2006, another study using a newer sleeping pill came up with similar results: Behavioral measures were more effective than the sleeping pills. Let's discuss some of these important tips for helping you get a good night's sleep so you feel refreshed in the morning.

⇨ Sleeping Tips

If you are having trouble getting to sleep, try the following suggestions, and/or try the CD meditation at the end of this chapter.

1. **Avoid caffeine** in the afternoon or evening. Caffeine can be found in coffee, chocolate, many sodas, and caffeinated teas. Certain medications, like decongestants, can cause insomnia in some people. (Speak with your doctor about other options for treating nasal congestion, if needed.) Alcohol sometimes helps with getting to sleep initially, but it may interfere with the quality of sleep and make it more likely that you will awaken in the middle of the night.
2. **Avoid heavy** meals right before bedtime.
3. **Regular exercise** is important and can help with sleep. However, it is best to avoid exercise in the two hours just before bed.
4. **If possible** use the bedroom only for activities such as sleep, meditation, and sex. Avoid eating, doing work activities, or talking on the phone in bed. It is helpful to have your body associate your bedroom with sleep.
5. **A regular** evening routine, such as taking a warm bath, meditating, or doing another relaxing activity, can help with sleep.
6. **Make your** bedroom dark, quiet, and a comfortable temperature.
7. **If you** tend to worry a lot, write your concerns on paper. Such a list can help prevent you from thinking about your problems again and again at night.

8. **Perhaps most** important, don't try too hard. If you try to go to sleep for 30 minutes and are still wide awake, get up from bed and do something else. It's useful to have a boring book on hand—something that you can get up and read (perhaps with a glass of warm skim milk) until you feel tired. Then go back to bed. Of course, one of the keys is picking a boring book, not a suspense novel. Alternatively, you might try reading a magazine article since it has a natural ending point.

9. **Try waking** up at the same time each morning and getting ready for bed at the same time every night. This schedule can help your body establish a rhythm. Establish a bedtime routine, such as brushing your teeth and taking a warm bath. However, after your regular bedtime routine, it is often best not to lie down in bed until you actually feel a little drowsy.

10. **If you** are having trouble sleeping, try a relaxation exercise. Use meditation to let go of those catastrophizing (and untrue) thoughts that just make the insomnia worse (like "I'll die without enough sleep," "I'll be useless tomorrow," "I'll never get to sleep"). Let go of your attempts to fall asleep and just focus on the current breath. Perhaps you can imagine your body sinking into the bed with each exhalation.

11. **Say you** have finally fallen asleep and someone or something wakes you up. What then? Well I can tell you what does not work. On occasion, someone has mistakenly called me at 3 a.m. Perhaps a nurse mistakenly thought I was the doctor on call for a problem. I have learned that it is a mistake to become increasingly annoyed by being awakened. Then it is tough to get back to sleep. What works a lot better is to handle the call (or whatever awakened me), roll over, and follow my breath. I quickly let go of thoughts about why I should

not have been called, or how I really need a full night's sleep, or how I will be a mess tomorrow. In other words, I nip my annoyance in the bud and get back to the breath.

12. **If, despite** these recommendations and despite trying the CD exercise below, you still are having problems with sleep, you can try a modest sleep restriction and then progressively increase the sleep duration. Set an alarm to wake up at the same time each morning. Even if you are tired, avoid napping during the day. If you think that your ideal amount of sleep to be refreshed is 8 hours, be ready to go to bed 7 hours before your time to get up. The next night, go to sleep 7½ hours before that time. And the following night, try going to bed 8 hours before that time.

⊙ Relaxation Meditation for Insomnia. Disk 2, Track 5. Length: 26 minutes.

When you have insomnia, put on this track and follow it. The exercise starts similarly to the guided meditation on CD 1. Later in the exercise, there is some guided imagery. When using this CD as a sleep aid, set the volume relatively low. Let go of your striving to fall asleep, and just listen to the instructions on the CD. If you get drowsy, feel free to turn the CD off. If you are still awake at the end of the meditation, spend another 20 minutes in quiet relaxation. If you are still having trouble sleeping, then go to your boring book and warm glass of milk.

Almost everyone has trouble sleeping on occasion. However, if your insomnia occurs frequently and does not improve with the above suggestions, you may want to discuss it with your doctor. Insomnia is sometimes caused by medical problems. For instance, an enlarged prostate may cause a man to wake up fre-

quently to urinate. Awakening with shortness of breath is a defi-
nite reason to seek a doctor's advice. Clinical depression and anxiety disorders may also cause insomnia and are described in
Chapter 16.

With sleep apnea, sleeping people may stop breathing for 10 to
20 seconds or more at a time. This apnea awakens them long
enough to get a breath. People with sleep apnea may wake up
over 100 times a night without being aware of it. Obviously, this
frequent awakening causes them considerable fatigue. They may
get morning headaches and high blood pressure as well. Usually,
but not always, people with sleep apnea are overweight and snore
loudly. Additionally, untreated sleep apnea increases the risk of
heart disease, so it is important for people with this problem to
seek medical attention.

Restless leg syndrome is another cause of insomnia. When people with this problem go to bed, their legs involuntarily kick and
move, waking up both themselves and sometimes their partners.
Several medications are useful in treating restless leg syndrome.

If you make the changes recommended in this chapter, both
your insomnia and your stress should decrease.

✎List changes to make in your sleep habits.

14

Change Your Environment

After working years as a nurse, Beverly had earned a promotion. It seemed like a good opportunity—better pay and more prestige as the head of a department. But during the two years she spent at the new job, she found herself becoming increasingly stressed and unhappy. With some further thought, she realized that the additional administrative responsibilities in her new job were keeping her from spending time with patients. Patient care was the part of nursing she really enjoyed. Returning to her old job was her most effective stress management technique.

Edith's husband physically abused her on a regular basis. As a result, she suffered from anxiety, depression, and a variety of other health problems. When she, with the help of community resources, left her abusive relationship, both her physical and her emotional health improved.

I KNOW I'VE been going on and on about reducing stress through internal changes like mindfulness, reframing, and keeping life in perspective. Yet, in many circumstances, like those in the examples above, external changes are *extremely* important. Sometimes, no amount of internal change is going to decrease your stress until you first deal with your external environment. If you are in the middle of the train tracks and the bullet train is aimed straight at you, it's really not the time for a sitting meditation!

Be careful, however, that you don't fall into the trap of always looking for an external solution. Abraham Maslow said, "When all you own is a hammer, every problem starts looking like a nail." If the only way you know how to deal with stress is to make external changes, you will make change after change. Eventually, you will find that you can never make enough external changes to be happy. It is always "I would be happy if only ___." Now that you have the screwdriver of mindfulness, the wrench of reframing, and the jigsaw of perspective, you can more wisely choose when to use your hammer of external change.

Stress can be a wake-up call—a signal to make changes or set new goals in your life. What are your dreams? Creating personal, financial, and spiritual goals and making plans to meet those goals are important. These goals and plans will help you manage your stress and achieve a full and exciting life.

❖ Goals Exercise

Take a moment now to think about what you would like improved in your life. What can you do to reach these goals and perhaps decrease the stress in your life?

I've encountered many people who improved their lives and decreased their stress by making important changes. External changes are not limited just to quitting a job or moving to a new town. The best change may be to stay at the same job, but to delegate, modify, or eliminate certain tasks. Frequently, people get stuck in inefficient practices. Being open to change is essential in managing stress and in doing well in your business and personal life.

✐ Changes List

Brainstorm possible changes you can make at home or work that might decrease your stress. Make sure the changes are concrete and can be realized.

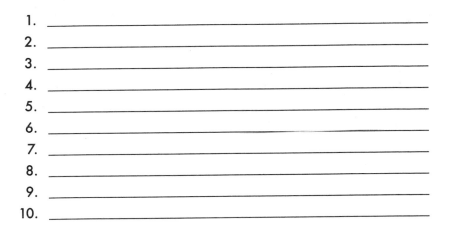

1. _____
2. _____
3. _____
4. _____
5. _____
6. _____
7. _____
8. _____
9. _____
10. _____

Go back through this list and place a "yes" if the change is definitely something you plan to do, a "no" if it is something you plan not to do, and a "?" if it would be best to think about it awhile.

Now that you've got a list of changes, it's time to make the game plan. You need to bring the changes from just ideas to reality. Make specific plans and set up a time line. If there is a big project, break it up into its component steps. Then, list a goal time to complete the step. If the goal is not met, all is not lost. You can learn from mistakes and reevaluate to make a new plan of action.

✐ Changes Game Plan

For each of the changes that you've determined should be made, fill out the table below (you may need to modify the table to fit your needs).

Change	Specific Steps Required for Change	Goal Date for Each Step
1.		
2.		
3.		
4.		

Now go ahead and put the specific tasks in your calendar or day planner. Ideally, take one small step in your plan right away.

If for some reason you don't meet a goal date, don't give up. Instead, just reassess. Remember, if a goal is not met, it isn't time to brand yourself a failure. Rather, it is time to ask what you learned from the attempt and then to make your second attempt wiser for the wear.

Another type of external strategy is to prepare reasonably for the future. Examples are

1. **Working** out finances for your basic needs, your children's education, and your retirement;

2. **Keeping** adequate insurance for you and your family;
3. **Discussing** family emergency plans (such as for fires, earth-quakes, or hurricanes, depending on where you live);
4. **Using** your seat belt and driving carefully;
5. **Wearing** a bicycle helmet when you're bicycling;
6. **Setting** up a good backup system for your computer (Is it obvious I learned a personal lesson on this one?);

When you take these precautions, you decrease your tendency to worry, and you also potentially prevent future stresses.

✒ Taking Precautions

Look at the above list of ways to take precautions for the future. What reasonable precautions would be wise for you? Please list them below and include specific plans to meet your goals.

1. _____
2. _____
3. _____
4. _____

15

Combine Strategies

The whole is more than the sum of its parts.

ARISTOTLE

THROUGHOUT THIS BOOK so far, we have discussed multiple strategies for dealing with stress. In our busy lives, might there be ways to combine these different strategies?

❖ Walking Combination

A regular practice of sitting meditation can be extremely effective in dealing with current stress and also in learning mindfulness. Regular exercise is also an important part of a healthy lifestyle and, in its own right, a very effective way to deal with stress. A walking meditation can combine both of these important activities. As you walk or jog, enjoy breathing the air and observe the sights and sounds in your environment. Consider saying to yourself a repetitive phrase or mantra that might consist of just counting "1, 2, 3, 4" with the inhalation and "1, 2, 3, 4" with the exhalation. Other options are to say something like "Peace" with the in breath and "Love" or "Smile" with the out breath. Or as we mentioned in an earlier chapter, you could use the mantra "Arrived" as you make each step (or every other step). If your thoughts drift, gently bring them back to the mantra. Alternatively, in this first part, you might focus on the sensations in your lower extremities, or you might do a choiceless awareness meditation as you walk.

After anywhere from 5 to 20 minutes of walking meditation, move to the next step of thinking about events and people for which you are grateful. As you stand tall, think to yourself something like "I am so grateful to have my son, Leo, in my life." Say it with conviction and visualize your child's face as you do this. Be grateful for what is directly around you in this present moment. You might say, "Thank you, God, for my ability to hear the birds singing." If you cannot hear, you might say, "I am very privileged to feel the wind and sun on my face." You might be thankful for and visualize some of the special moments of the week—perhaps a hug from a child, a special interaction with a friend, something going well at work, and so on. Some of the other areas for which you can express gratitude may include your basic necessities (like food and shelter), family, friends, work, health, or hobbies.

After 5 to 20 minutes devoted to gratefulness, start visualizing your plans for the day. Imagine how you will make your day go well. What might be exciting about the day? What challenges might the day bring? Visualize how you can meet those challenges. We do not have total control over our entire external environment. Situations may go as we plan or they may not. If something does not go as planned, resolve to learn from the process and not think of it as a failure. Visualize how you might use some of your stress management or communication techniques to deal confidently with any challenge that might happen today. At the end of the exercise, again note just a few things for which you are grateful, and congratulate yourself for setting aside time for yourself and your body. You may also spend some time during the walk silently repeating the loving-kindness or empathetic joy phrases mentioned in Chapter 11.

In summary: do a walking meditation, spend some time on gratitude, and then visualize the day. This type of combination can be used with other types of exercise, such as running or swimming. If you do this exercise first thing in the morning every morning (or most mornings), it will make an enormous difference in your life.

My life had become very busy. I had young twin boys and a busy practice. For some time, both my exercise regime and my sleep patterns suffered. I had started drinking two or three cups of coffee per day in order to compensate. In the long run, it seemed like a vicious circle. The coffee would help temporarily, but after the caffeine wore off, I sometimes felt worse and drank another cup. I resolved to wake up earlier in the morning (before the rest of the family was awake) and do a 25-minute run.

During the run, I would usually start meditating, then think about the things for which I was grateful, and then visualize how I could enjoy my day. I really enjoyed the routine. I stopped drinking coffee and actually felt much more energetic, even when I did not get many hours of sleep. Interestingly, I found that improving my posture by standing up straighter seemed to improve my energy level as well. I remembered my earlier injuries, so I avoided the mistake of starting with a five-mile run and instead kept to a shorter distance. Once in a while, I might swim instead, to give my legs a rest. In the meantime, I avoided evening television, so that I might get to bed earlier. In order to facilitate the early-morning jog, I would get everything ready the night before. Sometimes, I even wore my jogging shorts and a T-shirt to bed. I would try to iron my shirt and get my work clothes ready the night before, knowing that time in the morning might be tight.

Believe it or not, when I went to sleep, I looked forward to the run. One morning, the rest of my family woke up early, and my wife said, "Boys, how about a run with Dad?" So much for that time alone. However, flexibility is important. Not only did we have a great run with the baby jogger, but I still got my gratitude time . . . only it was better. I could share it with my sons. We talked together about all the things in life for which we were grateful. Not only did I focus my attention on gratitude, but hopefully I helped instill a great habit in my sons. Sometimes I would run on my own and sometimes with the boys. Either way, it was great (although running up a steep hill with two children in a baby jogger is no cakewalk).

Compared with running outside, I found swimming a relatively boring exercise. However, one week my left knee was really hurting. As opposed to just whining about my knee, I took it as an opportunity to do some cross-training and work on swimming. Often, when people swim they vary their routine to make it more interesting and to make the training more productive. For instance, they might do a few laps of crawl, a few of breaststroke, and a few of kick board. I decided that I would not only train my body by swimming but at the same time train my mind. I did so many laps of mantra meditation, so many laps of gratefulness, then laps of loving-kindness meditation, laps of planning for the day's challenges, laps of choiceless awareness meditation, and then threw in some more gratitude at the end. The swim was not boring; it was enjoyable. The time flew by, and at the end, both my body and my mind felt refreshed.

Remember, you would not expect to run a marathon without training your body. In order to live the most joyful life possible, you must train your mind.

Journaling

Occasionally, when a problem is on my mind, I get out my pen, or more often the computer, and write. Putting my thoughts on paper (or on my computer hard drive) decreases rumination and increases mindfulness. When all my concerns and points are on paper, I have less need to continually rehash them in my mind. Journaling also serves other functions, as discussed below.

Journaling Exercise

There are several ways to journal. You may start by listing whatever is on your mind. Avoid writing down what you should have done in a given situation. On the other hand, feel free to write down what you may have learned from an experience—what you might do differently next time. As you journal, use your stress management skills, such as: reframing, recognizing cognitive distortions and refuting them, and putting a situation in perspective. You can write about your goals and plans. You can plan how you might communicate with someone more effectively or how you might think of a situation differently. Some people like to write in a journal daily—some first thing in the morning and others at the end of their day. As we discussed in Chapter 8, listing things for which you are grateful is an important element of your writing.

Intimate Daily Devotions

This combination is especially useful for intimate/sexual relationships. Pamela Madison, founder of the Women's Sexuality Center in Santa Barbara, discusses a practice she calls "daily devotions." If you do not water your garden, the plants will likely die. If you do not nourish your sexual relationship, it may also suffer. We need to make time for each other, and that may be difficult in a family with multiple work and child-rearing commitments.

If you are in a relationship, during your daily devotions make 5 to 10 minutes of time together once or twice a day a priority. Usually, this is not a time for sexual intercourse to orgasm, but a time to connect. Often, in a marriage, there is a difference in libidos (sex drives). Making it clear that there is no expectation of orgasm during these sessions may make the partner with less libido feel less pressure and be more willing to participate.

During these sessions, the couple can try meditating together. One way is to focus on breathing together or on taking alternate breaths (as one partner inhales the other exhales and vice versa). The couple may then want to bring gratitude to the practice. Tell your partner what qualities in him or her you really appreciate physically, emotionally, and spiritually. Sexual play can often be part of the session; however, the goal is not orgasm.

Setting aside longer times for sex is important as well. Do not wait to be in the mood for your daily devotions or for your longer dates. Know that this time is essential for your and your partner's emotional and spiritual health.

In the longer sessions, orgasms will be more likely. However, even in the longer sessions, making the orgasm a goal may be counterproductive. If the goal is connection, both male and female orgasms are probably more likely, and the journey to get there may be much more enjoyable.

When the relationship is well nourished, the whole family benefits. If you are in a family with children, depending on their ages, you may need to set aside some time when your children are asleep, or if they are older, they might be able to play without you during the 5- to 10-minute daily devotions. Perhaps once a week, you might arrange babysitting or opt to take turns watching another family's children in order to have a longer period of intimacy.*

Don't wait to be in the mood to make love. Instead, make love to create the mood.

PAMELA MADISON

These three combinations have the potential to greatly improve your life: Making time every day for an exercise/meditation/gratitude exercise can make a huge difference in how you feel. Journaling can decrease stress in multiple ways. If you are in an intimate relationship, the daily devotions can significantly improve how you relate as a couple and how you feel about your relationship.

✎What ideas about combining strategies make sense for your life?

---

*If you are having problems with sexual function, your family doctor can be a good source of information (either for medication or for counseling referrals). Whenever there is a long pause during an office visit with a male patient, I know what the likely subject will be. Problems with sexual function are extremely common and are usually treatable.

16

When It's
More than Stress

He that won't be counseled can't be helped.
BENJAMIN FRANKLIN

One evening in the early 1980s, I was talking with a friend in a smoky bar. Suddenly, I felt an anxious urge to leave. At that time, I interpreted the feelings as claustrophobia. Several years later, I was in a house with a lot of animals and noticed similar feelings. My chest felt "tight," and it was difficult to breathe. My lung function was tested, and sure enough, it was significantly abnormal. I had asthma. That's likely what the tight anxious feeling had been years earlier.

ALTHOUGH THE MEDICAL conditions I will describe in this chapter are not the most common causes of anxiety, neither are they rare. One of the more frequent examples of a medical problem causing anxiety is hyperthyroidism; typical symptoms include a racing heartbeat, weight loss, anxiety, and a feeling of excessive warmth. Other signs of hyperthyroidism may include bulging of the eyes, enlargement of the thyroid gland (located in the front part of the neck), and an increase in the resting pulse rate.

In contrast to hyperthyroidism, in which the thyroid hormone level is high, in hypothyroidism the thyroid hormone level is low.

This problem tends to be associated with weight gain instead of weight loss, and it may also be associated with depression. I recently saw one woman who had been previously diagnosed as having postpartum depression. However, since the incidence of hypothyroidism is relatively high during the months following childbirth, I tested her for it. Indeed, she did have hypothyroidism. With replacement of the thyroid hormone, she felt much better, and the depression resolved.

If palpitations (racing or prominent heartbeat) are the most prevalent symptom of your anxiety, taking your pulse rate during the palpitations and discussing it with your doctor will help clarify the nature of the problem. See Figures 5 and 6 in Chapter 9 for instructions on taking your pulse. In general, a resting pulse rate between 50 and 100 that is regular in rhythm is not worrisome. An occasional early or late beat is usually not of concern. However, if your pulse is totally irregular or stays above 120 to 130 at rest, immediate medical attention is indicated. A pulse rate that is consistently between 100 and 120 at rest may be the result of anxiety, panic attacks, hyperthyroidism, or just being out of shape. If you have chest pain or shortness of breath with the palpitations, seek medical attention immediately.

Alcoholism and drug abuse are also associated with excessive amounts of anxiety. In addition, as we discussed earlier, caffeine and certain prescription and nonprescription medications can cause anxiety. Common offenders are decongestants, diet pills, and asthma medications. If you are on medication for diabetes, anxiety can result from your blood sugar's falling too low. Do not discontinue prescription medications without consulting your health care provider. Abrupt discontinuation of certain medications may also cause temporary anxiety and other more serious problems.

A few other extremely rare medical problems, such as non-cancerous adrenal tumors, can cause anxiety. Testing for these problems is necessary only in specific circumstances. (Such circumstances might include anxiety that is associated with very high blood pressure, a racing heart, headache, and feeling flushed.) Obviously, if the anxiety is associated with a symptom such as severe chest discomfort or shortness of breath, immediate medical attention is indicated.

The Anxiety Disorders

Excessive anxiety is more commonly caused by anxiety disorders than by the other medical conditions listed above. In fact, approximately 15 percent of the people in the United States have an anxiety disorder at some time in their lives. We all have stress, but when the anxiety is so severe that it significantly interferes with work or other aspects of your life, you may have an anxiety disorder. These disorders may be partially or fully a result of a shift in the normal biochemistry of the brain.

There are billions of nerve cells in the brain. Messages are transmitted down the length of an individual nerve cell by very small electrical impulses. Single nerve cells communicate with other nerve cells through chemical signals called *neurotransmitters*. Altered levels of these neurotransmitters contribute to anxiety disorders or clinical depression. A variety of medications can help with these disorders by regulating the levels of neurotransmitters. Many of these medications are not addictive. Potentially addictive medications may also be beneficial, when used carefully and with appropriate medical supervision.

People usually accept prescribed medication when they have been diagnosed with a medical problem such as diabetes or heart disease. However, some people with anxiety disorders or depression are reluctant to take medication. In people with diabetes, the pancreas does not produce sufficient insulin (or the cells are not sensitive to the insulin that is present); in some anxiety disorders or depression, the brain does not produce enough of a particular neurotransmitter (or perhaps the nerve cells are not sensitive enough to the amount of neurotransmitter that is present). For many people, nonpharmaceutical stress management techniques work well enough. However, people with severe anxiety disorders may need additional treatments.

Anxiety disorders and depression are medical conditions.* It should not be viewed as weakness to take medication for these problems, any more than it is weakness to take medication for diabetes. Diabetes can be treated with diet and exercise. However, when these changes alone are not effective enough, medication is also needed. In the same way, if the techniques you've read about in this book and/or counseling are not working well enough for an anxiety disorder, medication may be needed. It is important to treat these problems adequately for other reasons. Untreated, anxiety disorders and depression not only affect the people who have those conditions but also can dramatically affect their families and coworkers.

The burden of mental illness on health and productivity in the United States and throughout the world has long been underestimated. Data developed by the massive Global Burden of Disease study conducted by the World Health Organization, the World Bank, and Harvard University reveal that mental illness, including suicide, accounts for over 15 percent of the burden of disease in established market economies, such as the United States. This is more than the disease burden caused by all cancers.

NATIONAL INSTITUTE OF MENTAL HEALTH

---

*Depression here refers to clinical depression described further later in the chapter, not the occasional feelings of sadness that we all have.

Could untreated mental health problems cause other long-term difficulties? Research has shown that depressed people actually have shrinkage in an area of the brain called the hippocampus. Antidepressant medication seems to prevent that shrinkage. Mental health disorders fall into many different categories. For each type of disorder, there are effective types of medication and counseling.

Someone with a severe anxiety disorder may be immobilized. The anxiety may make functioning at work or at home impossible. Imagine you're driving along the freeway. Suddenly your heart starts racing, you feel as if you can't breathe, you are shaking, your chest feels uncomfortable, you feel numbness and tingling, and you have thoughts of death. Sound like fun? Hardly, but this may be a typical panic attack for people with panic disorder. Other symptoms may include dizziness, abdominal discomfort, nausea, sweating, choking, flushing, feelings of entrapment, and fears of going crazy or out of control. These attacks often happen for no apparent reason. Sometimes, the attacks are so frightening that people develop a fear of going out of the house (a condition called *agoraphobia*) because they worry that they might have an attack while out. Panic attacks, like the other disorders we will discuss, are very treatable with counseling and/or medication (often, a combination of both is most appropriate).

Phobias are exaggerated fears of a specific object or situation. Examples are claustrophobia (fear of closed spaces), fear of high places, and fear of flying. These problems are often alleviated with a short bit of counseling. If someone is scared of flying, they might practice a relaxation exercise while imagining being on a plane. Later, they might try the exercise while in an airport, and then when actually on a plane. However, if you have an extreme fear of flying and take only one plane trip per year, it may be helpful to take antianxiety medication at the beginning of the flight.

People with obsessive-compulsive disorder, or OCD, are bothered and even disabled by their obsessions and compulsions. Obsessions are recurrent or persistent thoughts that become intrusive. People with these disorders are so disturbed by these thoughts or ideas that they may feel compelled to do certain actions. For instance, they may have recurrent thoughts of being contaminated, compelling them to wash their hands excessively (perhaps even hundreds of times a day). Other obsessions may involve feelings of aggression or of losing control. We have all double-checked that a door is locked or that the stove is turned off. However, in OCD, this checking behavior may be excessive. This condition may also be improved with medication and behavioral counseling.

The term *generalized anxiety disorder* refers to excessive anxiety throughout the day as opposed to the intermittent nature of the anxiety in panic disorder. Social phobia is a persistent fear of certain social situations, such as an immobilizing fear of talking in front of others or of eating in front of others.

Posttraumatic stress disorder (PTSD) became well known after the Vietnam War. This disorder occurs following a traumatic event that is outside the range of normal human experience. Examples of such traumatic events are war experiences and other violent episodes, such as being raped or witnessing a murder. Some of the more common symptoms of PTSD include: having recurring or intrusive recollections of the event, having recurrent disturbing dreams, and being startled easily.

In addition to anxiety disorders, a common medical problem is clinical depression. This is different from occasionally being down or "depressed." In clinical depression, the depressed mood occurs very frequently, for at least two weeks. Activities that formerly brought enjoyment cease to do so or are abandoned entirely. A clinical depression often brings a change in appetite, weight loss or gain, fatigue, and decreased concentration. Other common symptoms are insomnia (especially early-morning awakening with trouble getting back to sleep), trouble concentrating, feelings of worthlessness, excessive guilt, and recurrent thoughts of death.

If you have recurrent thoughts of suicide or if anyone you know starts talking about suicide, immediately seek professional attention. Do not ignore these statements. If you do not know of a professional to call, call telephone information (411) for a suicide hotline or call 911. Pay attention if someone starts saying good-byes or starts giving away prized possessions. Clinical depression may include feelings of hopelessness and thoughts of never improving. Although depressed people often feel as if their condition will never improve, the vast majority do improve, given time and the appropriate treatments. In these cases, suicide is truly a permanent solution to a temporary problem.

Both environmental and genetic factors contribute to anxiety disorders and depression. Why are some people more likely than others to develop depression? One study found that people who had a variation in one particular gene were indeed more likely to develop depression when experiencing a given stressful life event.

Seasonal affective disorder, or SAD, is a depression prominent in the winter months. This disorder may respond to specifically designed lights. Not infrequently, women experience increased sadness or anxiety after having a baby. This condition is termed *postpartum depression* and may be caused by both the dramatic hormonal shifts and the social changes that occur after delivering a baby. Postpartum depression is a temporary condition and usually responds to support groups, counseling, and/or medication.* Premenstrual syndrome (PMS) includes excessive anxiety, depression,

---

*As mentioned earlier, thyroid disorders are also not uncommon after delivery and are readily treatable if identified. They may also cause depression and/or anxiety.

and possibly other symptoms such as breast swelling in the days preceding a woman's period. PMS responds to regular exercise and good nutrition, but in more severe cases, medications such as antidepressants are very useful. Dysthymia is a low-grade depression, and the best treatment for it is somewhat controversial. The treatment might include counseling, antidepressants, or even an herbal preparation called *hypericum* (St. John's Wort).*

In bipolar disorder (or manic depressive illness), feelings of depression alternate with "manic" states. (Symptoms of mania may include elation, irritability, racing thoughts, increased energy, staying up all night, grandiosity, pressured speech, and irrational activity.)

A disorder that has received recent recognition is adult attention deficit disorder. Attention deficit disorder (ADD) first appears in children who have trouble concentrating in class. Some, but not all, of these children are "hyperactive." When children with ADD become adults, their symptoms may or may not continue. Adults with ADD may have trouble concentrating and staying focused on a task.

If you believe that you, or someone you know, may have one of these disorders, discuss the issue with a health professional. Appropriate professionals include your family doctor, your internist, or a psychiatrist. Counselors, psychologists, and other qualified therapists may also be helpful, but if medications are needed, you will have to talk with a medical doctor.

While he was participating in my stress management class, Daniel's stress level significantly improved. Additionally, as he

---

*It is best to consult with your health care provider before taking this or certain other herbal products. Many herbal products, such as hypericum, have potential side effects and significant drug interactions.

reviewed the class notes, he recognized that, for many years, he had experienced several of the symptoms associated with a clinical depression. He frequently suffered from fatigue, insomnia, decreased sex drive, and a variety of vague physical complaints. He had trouble concentrating and frequently felt sad. He realized that these symptoms had been present to one extent or another for many years. Although the techniques he learned in the class helped, he still felt sad much of the time.

For some reason, Daniel had previously seen this sadness as a sign of weakness. Even upon learning about the medical syndrome of depression, he was reluctant to seek treatment. Finally, he decided that life was too short for him not to do what he could to feel better. He went to see his family doctor, who recommended that he start both an antidepressant medication and counseling. Daniel was not having much improvement after six weeks on the antidepressant. His doctor, however, was not discouraged, since he knew that there were perhaps 20 antidepressants on the market.

Daniel was switched to another antidepressant and, after being on the treatment for approximately one month, noticed a dramatic change in how he felt. The fatigue, insomnia, loss of sex drive, sadness, poor concentration, and physical symptoms were all decreased. He finally felt like himself again and wondered why he had waited so long to seek treatment.

Dora was 61 years old and had had a problem with anxiety since the fourth grade; she had started having panic attacks at the age of 12. She had been through multiple medications and seen many psychiatrists and counselors. She had had some relief with the relaxation techniques that she had learned, along with a relatively small dose of a benzodiazepine (a type of tranquilizer).

Still, she was so bothered by panic attacks and agoraphobia that she would not drive.

In general, doctors avoid prescribing too much of the benzo-diazepine class of medicine, since they are potentially addictive. However, if used carefully, they can be very beneficial. (Sometimes, we prescribe the benzodiazepines short-term as we wait for the nonaddictive medications to "kick in.") In Dora's case, I felt she was not getting adequate medication. I increased the total dose of benzodiazepine and, at the same time, started her on a new antidepressant that is generally effective for anxiety after it has had some time to kick in.

I saw Dora two weeks later, and she was amazed. She felt the best she had felt in a long time. She was peaceful throughout the day and could sleep at night. She felt "in control" and "ready to venture out." Putting it simply, she said, "I just feel good." This woman, who had suffered from a severe anxiety disorder for half a century, finally felt well. Prior to starting on the new medications, she had said she was "at the end of her rope" and had even thought about suicide.

Sometimes, a person's biochemical abnormality is too great for counseling or stress management techniques alone. Sometimes, medication is needed to help temporarily—long enough for someone to learn the techniques and gain confidence in his or her ability to deal with anxiety. Dora's message to others was "If you need help with medication, by all means, get help. If the first medicine does not work, don't be discouraged. Keep trying until you find something that does work." Interestingly, as Dora reviewed this book and CD set and continued to practice the mindfulness techniques, her need for medication decreased. Previously, she had tried to analyze why she was having her thoughts of panic. She learned an alternative: As soon as she noticed the nonproductive thoughts, she gently let them go. She was surprised to find that her panic did not last hours. Instead, it never fully developed, and the milder anxiety lasted only about 30 seconds.

Do not get me wrong; I am not a "pills-for-everyone" doctor. The vast majority of people do very well without anxiety medication. In fact, as the below story illustrates, many people are prescribed these medicines prematurely.

Angela was depressed and anxious and didn't want to get out of bed in the mornings. A previous doctor had prescribed an antidepressant. Angela did not like how she felt on the medication, so she stopped it. When Angela visited me, she revealed that she was working her way through college. She spent 15 hours a week in class and needed to study another 15 hours a week. In order to make ends meet financially, she had taken a job that initially required an additional 20 to 25 hours of work a week. She was doing fine until her boss asked Angela to do a little more work here and there. Before Angela knew it, in addition to her schoolwork, she was working 40 to 50 hours a week at her job—and she was miserable.

At our visit, instead of my jumping to prescribe another antidepressant, we brainstormed on how she could reduce her work hours. We discussed assertiveness skills and ways she could approach her boss to decrease her stress and improve her health.

As you can see, we should not rely on medications to cure all our ills. That is one of the very reasons that I wrote this book: to give people a wide variety of nondrug options to deal with stress and anxiety. However, some people do need medications, and for those people, we must remove any stigma associated with the drugs. When the medications are used, they should be used in conjunction with, and not instead of, stress management techniques. All medications, including antidepressants and antianxiety medications, have potential risks and side effects. A good health care practitioner can help you weigh the risks and benefits and will closely monitor your progress.

If you have high blood pressure that is not controlled with diet and exercise, take medication before you have a heart attack or stroke. If you have clinical depression or an anxiety disorder and do not get adequate relief with stress management techniques and counseling, seek further help.

17

Conclusion

Education is not the filling of a pail, but the lighting of a fire.

WILLIAM BUTLER YEATS

IN THIS BOOK, I have introduced to you a number of techniques you can use to manage the stress in your life. By reading this book and practicing the techniques that I have suggested, you are taking an active role in acquiring a happier and healthier life for yourself and for those around you.

Whatever stressful events you may encounter throughout your life, remember the importance of bringing yourself back to the present moment. Enjoy your life and your family, friends, and coworkers. Enjoy the next breath and feel the ground with each step. You do not need to clear your mind to have peace of mind; just enjoy that very next moment and pay keen attention to each sensation. Enjoy breathing, walking, eating, driving, showering, washing the dishes, and petting your dog.

Stress management is a lifelong practice. We frequently need to be reminded of stress management techniques. In that light, I encourage you to review selected chapters in this book and the CDs as needed. Additionally, use the list of books and Web sites at the end of this book to further explore stress management techniques.

As you continue your journey in learning, your knowledge will advance both intellectually and experientially. As your studies and experiences continue, you may find that information you understood on a relatively superficial level becomes understood on a deeper level. Sometimes, these insights are sudden, and other times, they develop over time. Through it all, continue the journey of learning with that fire of curiosity.

This journey that began with the goal of stress management is really a journey that brings you to the core of what life is about. We do not want to get to our death and find that we have never really lived. May that idea also encourage your fire of learning to burn brightly and joyously.

Realize that this learning you do is not just for yourself. It is for your family, friends, work associates, and community. Each time you respond with less stress and more compassion, the ripples of your actions extend in ways you may never know. A small bit of kindness may change how another feels and acts, and so on and so on down the line. With global communication taking place by way of the Internet, over the phone, and in person thanks to air travel, a small act of compassion for your next-door neighbor may positively impact people on the other side of the world. In these times of hostility and violence, peace must begin within our own selves. Only then can these small ripples of compassion extend and create a more peaceful world. Certainly that goal should also stoke your fire to learn and continue this very important journey.

May you have peace and happiness,
and may your friends, family, and all of us
have peace and happiness.

SUGGESTED READING LIST

General Stress Management and Health

The Healthy Mind, Healthy Body Handbook by David S. Sobel and Robert Ornstein. Los Altos, CA: DRx, 1996.

The Wellness Book: The Comprehensive Guide to Maintaining Health and Treating Stress-Related Illness by Herbert Benson and Eileen M. Stuart. New York: Simon & Schuster, 1992.

Don't Sweat the Small Stuff by Richard Carlson. New York: Hyperion, 1997.

Minding the Body, Mending the Mind by Joan Borysenko. New York: Bantam Books, 1987.

Stressed Is Desserts Spelled Backward by Brian Luke Seaward. Berkeley, CA: Conari Press, 1999.

Managing Stress: Principles for Health and Well-Being, 5th ed., by Brian Luke Seaward. Sudbury, MA: Jones & Bartlett, 2006.

General Stress Management, Emphasizing Review of Research

Mind/Body Health: The Effects of Attitudes, Emotions, and Relationships, 3rd ed., by Brent Q. Hafen, Keith J. Karren, Kathryn J. Frandsen, and N. Lee Smith. San Francisco: Benjamin Cummings, 2005.

Mindfulness

Peace Is Every Step by Thich Nhat Hahn. New York: Bantam Books, 1991.

Full Catastrophe Living by Jon Kabat-Zinn. New York: Dell, 1990.

Wherever You Go There You Are: Mindfulness Meditation in Everyday Life by Jon Kabat-Zinn. New York: Hyperion, 1994.

Insight Meditation: A Step-By-Step Course on How to Meditate by Sharon Salzberg and Joseph Goldstein. Boulder, CO: Sounds True, 2001.

Coming to Our Senses by Jon Kabat-Zinn. New York: Hyperion, 2005.

Meditation for Beginners by Jack Kornfield. Boulder, CO: Sounds True, 2004.

Cognitive Therapy

Feeling Good by David Burns. New York: Avon Books, 1980.

Type A Personality

Treating Type A Behavior and Your Heart by Meyer Friedman and Diane Ulmer. New York: Ballantine Books, 1984.

Lifestyle

Simplify Your Life by Elaine St. James. New York: Hyperion, 1994.

Margin and *The Overload Syndrome* (these books are available together, in quite small print, or individually) by Richard Swenson. Colorado Springs, CO: Navpress, 2002.

Healthy Pleasures by Robert Ornstein and David Sobel. New York: Addison-Wesley, 1989.

Communication

Messages: The Communication Skills Book by Matthew McKay, Martha Davis, and Patrick Fanning. Oakland, CA: New Harbinger, 1995.

The Basics of Nonviolent Communication by Marshall Rosenberg. DVD available at www.cnvc.org.

Work-Related Stress

Don't Sweat the Small Stuff at Work by Richard Carlson. New York: Hyperion, 1998.

The Truth about Burnout by Christina Maslach and Michael P. Leiter. San Francisco: Jossey-Bass, 1997.

Relationships and Stress

Don't Sweat the Small Stuff with Your Family by Richard Carlson. New York: Hyperion, 1998.

Love and Survival by Dean Ornish. New York: HarperCollins, 1998.

Anxiety Disorders

The Anxiety Book by Jonathan Davidson and Henry Dreher. New York: Penguin Putnam, 2003.

Panic Disorder

Don't Panic by R. Reid Wilson. New York: HarperCollins, 1996.

Depression

Understanding Depression by Raymond J. DePaulo and Leslie Ann Horvitz. Hoboken, NJ: Wiley, 2002.

The Mindful Way through Depression: Freeing Yourself from Chronic Unhappiness by J. Mark Williams, John D. Teasdale, Zindel Segal, and Jon Kabat-Zinn. New York: Guilford Press, 2007.

Mindfulness-Based Cognitive Therapy for Depression: a New Approach to Preventing Relapse by Zindel Segal, Mark Williams, and John Teasdale. New York: Guilford Press, 2002.

Logotherapy/Importance of Purpose

Man's Search for Meaning by Victor Frankl. New York: Simon & Schuster, 1959.

Time Management

Getting Things Done: The Art of Stress Free Productivity by David Allen. New York: Penguin Books, 2001.

Raising Children

Setting Limits with Your Strong-Willed Child: Eliminating Conflict by Establishing Clear, Firm and Respectful Boundaries by Robert MacKenzie. New York: Random House, 2001.

How to Talk So Kids Will Listen and Listen So Kids Will Talk by Adele Faber and Elaine Mazlish. New York: Avon Books, 1980.

Everyday Blessings: The Inner Work of Mindful Parenting by Myla and Jon Kabat-Zinn. New York: Hyperion, 1997.

Raising Children Compassionately by Marshall Rosenberg. Encinitas, CA: PuddleDancer Press, 2005.

Spirituality and Compassion

A Path with Heart: A Guide through the Perils and Pitfalls of Spiritual Life by Jack Kornfield. New York: Bantam Books, 1993.

After the Ecstasy, the Laundry by Jack Kornfield. New York: Bantam Books, 2000.

One Dharma by Joseph Goldstein. New York: HarperCollins, 2003.

RECOMMENDED WEB SITES

Important information on stress, including updates about this book and my
   related work: www.stressremedy.com.
Finding a mindfulness-based stress reduction teacher: www.umassmed
   .edu/cfm/mbsr/.
Finding a counselor specializing in anxiety disorders: www.adaa.org/Getting
   Help/FindATherapist.asp.
Information on nonviolent communication: www.cnvc.org.
Meditation retreats: www.spiritrock.org and www.dharma.org.
Mindful eating: www.tcme.org.

CD CONTENTS

Disk 1

Tracks:
   Six-Minute Meditation
   Guided Meditation
   Letting Go Meditation
   Sound, Breath, Body, Thoughts & Emotions
   Walking Meditation

Disk 2

Tracks:
   Eating Meditation
   Stretching Meditation
   Letting Go and Reframing Exercise
   Loving-Kindness Meditation
   Relaxation Exercise for Insomnia

NOTES

Introduction

xiv *Than people with normal stress* Richard Shulz and Scott Beach, "Caregiving as a Risk Factor for Mortality." *Journal of the American Medical Association,* Vol. 282, 1999; pp. 2215–2219.

xiv *Aging 9 to 17 years.* Elissa Epel, Elizabeth, et al., "Accelerated Telomere Shortening in Response to Life Stress," *Proceedings of the National Academy of Sciences,* Vol. 101, No. 49, December 7, 2004, pp. 17312–17315.

xiv *72 percent increased risk of stroke.* Susan Everson et al., "Stress-Induced Blood Pressure Reactivity and Incident Stroke in Middle-Aged Men," *Stroke,* Vol. 32, 2001, pp. 1263–1270.

xiv *Stress as you read these words.* "Americans Engage in Unhealthy Behaviors to Manage Stress," American Psychological Association press release, February 23, 2006.

xvi *97 percent of physicians are aware.* http://www.epocrates.com/landing/survey/stress.html?cid=EMN1107.

xx *Number one impediment to academic success.* American College Health Association–National College Health Assessment (ACHA-NCHA), Web summary, updated April 2006. Available at http://www.acha.org/projects_programs/ncha_sampledata.cfm.

xx *Dying from heart disease and stroke.* Mika Kivimaka et al., "Work Stress and Risk of Cardio Vascular Mortality: Prospective Cohort of Industrial Employees," *British Medical Journal,* Vol. 325, No. 857, October 19, 2002, p. 857; and Corine Aboa-Éboulé et al., "Job Strain and Risk of Acute Recurrent Coronary Heart Disease Events," *Journal of the American Medical Association,* Vol. 298, No. 14, pp. 1652–1660.

xx *Those who did no stress management.* James Blumenthal et al., "Stress Management and Exercise Training in Cardiac Patients with Myocardial Ischemia," *Archives of Internal Medicine,* Vol. 157, 1997, pp. 2213–2223.

xx *The risk of Alzheimer's disease.* R. S. Wilson, "Proneness to Psychological Distress Is Associated with Risk of Alzheimer's Disease," *Neurology,* Vol. 61, No. 11, December 2003, pp. 1479–1485; and R. S. Wilson, "Proneness to Psychology Distress and Risk of Alzheimer's Disease in a Biracial Community," *Neurology,* Vol. 64, No. 2, pp. 380–382.

xx *Workers under high levels of stress.* Steven Sauter et al., "Stress at Work," National Institute for Occupational Safety and Health (NIOSH), U.S. Department of Health and Human Services (DHHS), Publication No. 99–101. DHHS (NIOSH) Web site: http://www.cdc.gov/niosh/stresswk.html.

3. Learn to Relax

9 *Softens your hyperalertness.* Herbert Benson and Miriam Z. Klipper, *The Relaxation Response.* New York: Harper Torch, 2000 (initial version in 1975).

10 *A 23 percent decreased chance of dying.* Robert Schneider et al., "Long-Term Effects of Stress Reduction on Mortality in Persons ≥55 Years of Age with Systemic Hypertension," *American Journal of Cardiology,* Vol. 95, May 1, 2005, pp. 1060–1064.

10 *Important structural changes in the brain.* S. W. Lazar et al., "Meditation Experience Is Associated with Increased Cortical Thickness," *Neuroreport,* Vol. 16, No. 17, November 28, 2005, pp. 1893–1897.

18 *". . .present moment—wonderful moment."* Thich Nhat Hahn, *Present Moment Wonderful Moment.* Berkeley, CA: Parallax Press, 1990, p. 32.

18 *Remember additional feelings of wellness.* Herbert Benson and Marg Stark, *Timeless Healing.* New York: Fireside, 1997.

4. Learn to Enjoy Your Day

32 *Washing one dish at a time.* Thich Nhat Hanh, *Peace Is Every Step.* New York: Bantam Books, 1991, pp. 26–27.

5. Put Mindfulness into Practice

41 *Reminders of mindfulness.* Thich Nhat Hanh, *Peace Is Every Step.* New York: Bantam Books, 1991, pp. 18–20.

48 *As a guide from beyond—RUMI.* Printed with permission of Maypop and Coleman Barks from *Say I Am You: Poetry Interspersed with Stories of Rumi and Shams by Rumi,* translated by John Moyne and Coleman Barks. Athens, GA: Maypop, 1994, p. 41.

56 *Feelings into words helps reduce distress.* Matthew D. Lieberman et al., "Putting Feelings into Words: Affect Labeling Disrupts Amygdala Activity in Response to Affective Stimuli," *Psychological Science,* Vol. 18, May 2007, pp. 421–428.

57 *Mindfulness-based cognitive therapy, or MBCT.* Zindel Segal, Mark Williams, and John Teasdale, *Mindfulness-Based Cognitive Therapy for Depression: A New Approach to Preventing Relapse.* New York: Guilford Press, 2002.

6. Change Your Thoughts

70 *Nine categories of cognitive distortion.* David D. Burns, *Feeling Good.* New York: Avon Books, 1980, pp. 42–43.

79 *Child as an "experiential learner."* Robert MacKenzie, *Setting Limits with Your Strong-Willed Child: Eliminating Conflict by Establishing Clear, Firm and Respectful Boundaries.* New York: Random House, 2001.

82 *Visualization you can use to help.* Jack Kornfield, *A Path with Heart.* New York: Bantam Books, 1993, p. 165.

7. Slow Down

89 *Higher risk of heart disease.* Friedman admits to an upholsterer's pointing out the excessive wear but claims that the revelation about the type A personality did not occur until a little later. Meyer Friedman and Diane Ulmer, *Type A Behavior and Your Heart.* New York: Ballantine Books, 1984.

90 *Risk of developing a heart problem.* I. Kawachi, D. Sparrow, A. Spiro, et al., "A Prospective Study of Anger and Coronary Heart Disease: The Normative Aging Study," *Circulation,* Vol. 94, 1996, pp. 2090–2095.

90 *Risk of high blood pressure.* Lijing Lan et al., "Psychosocial Factors and Risk of Hypertension and Coronary Artery Risk Development in Young Adults (CARDIA) Study," *Journal of the American Medical Association,* Vol. 290, 2003, pp. 2138–2148.

92 *Difficult life of medical residents.* Samuel Shem, *The House of God.* New York: Dell Books, 1981.

8. Keep Life in Perspective

100 *Making a "gratitude journal."* Sarah Ban Breathnach, *Simple Abundance.* New York: Warner Books, 1995.

105 *Volunteered at least once a week.* Brent Q. Hafen, Keith J. Karren, Kathryn J. Frandsen, and N. Lee Smith, *Mind/Body Health.* Boston: Allyn & Bacon, 1996, p. 403.

105 *"If you're alive, it isn't."* Richard Bach, *Illusions: The Adventures of a Reluctant Messiah.* New York: Dell, 1997, p. 159.

107 *React in a similar scenario.* "30 Ideas to Reduce Stress." Available at www.thriveonline.com/health/stress.30tips.html.

108 *JOHN-ROGER WILLIAMS.* John-Roger Williams and Peter McWilliams, *You Can't Afford the Luxury of a Negative Thought.* Los Angeles: Prelude Press, p. 277.

111 *He trips or falls down.* A. H. Benjamin and Tim Warnes, *It Could Have Been Worse.* Waukesha, WI: Little Tiger Press. 1999.

9. Improve Your Lifestyle

122 *"Almost every day of the year."* Richard Carlson, *Don't Sweat the Small Stuff with Your Family.* New York: Hyperion, 1998, p. 25.

123 *That comes across our desks.* David Allen, *Getting Things Done: The Art of Stress Free Productivity.* New York: Penguin Books, 2001.

123 *Keeping stress in check.* Robert Ornstein and David Sobel, *Healthy Pleasures.* Reading, MA: Addison-Wesley, 1989.

124 *A recent study.* University of Nottingham (2007, December 3). "Happiness Comes Cheap—Even For Millionaires," *ScienceDaily.* Retrieved December 4, 2007, from http://www.sciencedaily.com/releases/2007/11/071130224158.htm.

126 *Over 50,000 women.* Frank B. Hu, Tricia Y. Li, Graham A. Colditz, Walter C. Willett, and JoAnn E. Manson, "Television Watching and

Other Sedentary Behaviors in Relation to Risk of Obesity and Type 2 Diabetes Mellitus in Women," *Journal of the American Medical Association,* Vol. 289, 2003, pp. 1785–1791.

135 *Obesity and insulin resistance.* Damien McNamara, "Regular Breakfast Eaters at Lower Risk for Obesity," *Family Practice News,* May 15, 2003, p. 10.

138 *Increased resistance to colds.* Sheldon Cohen et al., "Social Ties and Susceptibility to the Common Cold," *Journal of the American Medical Association,* Vol. 277, No. 24, June 25, 1997, pp. 1940–1945.

138 *To a longer life.* J. S. House, K. R. Landis, and D. Umberson, "Social Relationships and Health," *Science,* Vol. 241, 1988, p. 545.

138 *Incidence of heart disease.* Eugene Braunwald (Ed.), *Heart Disease: A Textbook of Cardiovascular Medicine,* 16th ed. New York: W. B. Saunders, 2001, pp. 2247–2248.

10. Improve Your Communication

144 *"My grandchildren, in this same way."* Carl Rogers, *A Way of Being.* Boston: Houghton Mifflin, 1980, pp. 22–23.

153 *Motivation, she felt better.* Adapted from a story by mediator Judith Rubenstein.

159 *"Take your time."* Marshall Rosenberg, *Raising Children Compassionately.* Encinitas, CA: PuddleDancer Press, 2005, pp. 9–10.

161 *Determined by nonverbal cues.* Albert Mehrabian and Susan R. Ferris, "Inference of Attitudes from Nonverbal Communication in Two Channels," *Journal of Consulting Psychology,* Vol. 31, No. 3, June 1967, pp. 248–258.

11. Deal with Anger and Frustration

169 *Increased risk of heart disease.* Eugene Braunwald (Ed.), *Heart Disease: A Textbook of Cardiovascular Medicine,* 16th ed. New York: W. B. Saunders, 2001; pp. 2244–2245.

169 *"Take my mind as well?"* Jon Kabat-Zinn, *Wherever You Go, There You Are.* New York: Hyperion, 1994, p. 49.

174 *Other ways of dealing with anger.* The Dalai Lama and Howard C. Cutler, *The Art of Happiness.* New York: Riverhead Books, 1998, Chapter 10.

13. Improve Your Sleep

191 *Given the behavioral treatments.* C. Morin et al., "Behavioral and Pharmacological Therapies for late-life insomnia: A randomized controlled trial," *Journal of the American Medical Association,* Vol. 281, March 19, 1999, pp. 991–999.

191 *More effective than the sleeping pills.* B. Siversten et al., "Cognitive Behavioral Therapy vs. Zopiclone for the Treatment of Chronic Primary Insomnia in Older Adults: A Randomized Controlled Trial," *Journal of the American Medical Association,* Vol. 295, June 28, 2006, pp. 2851–2858.

15. Combine Strategies

207 *She calls "daily devotions."* The Women's Sexuality Center Web site is www.womensexualitycenter.com.

16. When It's More than Stress

213 *At some time in their lives.* R. Michels and P. M. Marzuk, "Progress in Psychiatry," *New England Journal of Medicine,* Vol. 13, No. 2, 1993; pp. 11–18.

215 *Seems to prevent that shrinkage.* Y. Sheline et al., "Untreated Depression and Hippocampal Volume Loss," *American Journal of Psychiatry,* Vol. 160, 2003, pp. 1516–1518.

217 *A given stressful life event.* A. Caspi et al., "Influence of Life Stress on Depression: Moderation by a Polymorphism in the 5-HTT Gene," *Science,* Vol. 327, July 5, 2003, pp. 28–29.

ACKNOWLEDGMENTS

I owe a debt of gratitude to the following people: First and foremost, I would like to thank my wonderful wife, Dana, who has provided me with love, support, and a lot of excellent advice. My children, Samuel and Zachary, inspire me and continually teach me about life and love.

My parents, Shirley and Seymour Winner, and my sister, Jody Ginsberg, all helped provide a wonderful, loving environment for me to grow up in and continued to offer support and love over the years.

I'd like to offer special thanks to my patients and students, who have taught me so much, and thanks to a variety of authors whose wisdom has been made available to me and others.

I very much appreciate the invaluable inspiration and help provided by my friends. And thank you to the people at Da Capo, including Matthew Lore and Courtney Napoles, and to my agent, Stephany Evans, for believing in the project and helping it come to fruition.

Rowan Jacobsen deserves special thanks for his expertise in helping with the writing. His ideas helped to both strengthen the introduction and make other sections of the book more interactive and readable. Don Ollis of A Room with a Vu did an excellent job with the CD recording and editing. Thanks to my copy editor, Margaret Ritchie, and the project editor, Renee Caputo. Susan Myers's technical drawings really enhance the book. Michael Weiser (www.photoperception.com) and Clint Weisman did the photography for my Web site, www.stressremedy.com. Some editorial review was also done by Donna Beech and Joyce Anne Grabel (www.editorialdirectionllc.com). Thank you to my superb coworkers and colleagues at Sansum Clinic, including my office partner and friend, Kari Mathison, who lent a patient ear during the development of the book.

I also owe a debt of gratitude to the people who reviewed the book for comments and/or endorsements. Motivated by their shared vision of helping people deal with stress more effectively, they offered thoughtful suggestions and important comments. They include Alexander Bystritsky, Richard Roberts, Bruce Bagley, Laura Richardson Roberts, David Zajano, Steve Shearer, Larry Bascom, Lynn Matis, Mike Lawson, M. Greg Stathakis, Nancy Murdock, Diana Winston, Jack Kornfield, Jack Canfield, and Dean Ornish.

INDEX